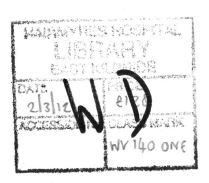

T. Metin Önerci

Diagnosis in Otorhinolaryngology

T. Metin Önerci

Diagnosis in Otorhinolaryngology

With 432 Figures and 62 Tables

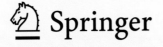 Springer

Prof. T. Metin Önerci
Hacettepe University
Faculty of Medicine
Dept. of Otorhinolaryngology
06100 Ankara
Sihhiya
Turkey
metin@tr.net

ISBN: 978-3-642-00498-8   e-ISBN: 978-3-642-00499-5

DOI: 10.1007/978-3-642-00499-5

Springer Dordrecht Heidelberg London New York

Library of Congress Control Number: 2009926009

© Springer-Verlag Berlin Heidelberg 2009

Cover design: eStudioCalamar, Figueres/Berlin

Printed on acid-free paper

Springer is part of Springer Science+Business Media (www.springer.com)

Preface

In preparing the material for this book, I took the advice of my students who generously shared their views and opinions with me. I was told that it would be preferable to have images of the various diseases with legends describing the disease. Students would be able to learn and retain the information more successfully if the material was accompanied by pictures and schematic drawings.

Recent advances in technology have made it possible to photograph regions that are difficult to view with the naked eye, such as the ear, nose, throat, nasopharynx, and larynx – all the areas of otorhinolaryngology. Such an illustrated text in this field is important and necessary for teaching purposes.

In this book I tried to compile images of the basic conditions that are commonly seen in general practice and to give the reader a visual survey with a brief description of the condition. I added tables and schematic drawings in order to provide practical information. It is not the purpose of this book to be a comprehensive textbook, since many textbooks are already available with more detailed information of the conditions illustrated here.

This book is primarily intended for medical students, family and general practitioners, and ENT trainees. It may also serve as basic reading material for those in allied specialties. I hope my colleagues find this book useful and it contributes toward their teaching purposes.

I would like to thank Ebru Oralli, the illustrator, who drew all the illustrations; my colleagues for their very kind help in the preparation of this book; and the staff of Springer-Verlag for their valuable assistance during the publication process.

Ankara, Turkey   T. Metin Önerci

Contents

EAR

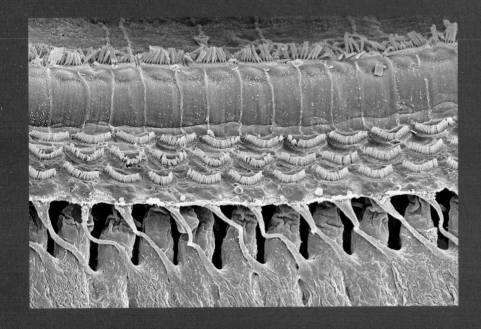

CONTENTS

T. Metin Önerci: *Diagnosis in Otorhinolaryngology*
DOI: 10.1007/978-3-642-00499-5_1, © Springer-Verlag Berlin Heidelberg 2009

1.1

Ear Anatomy

a

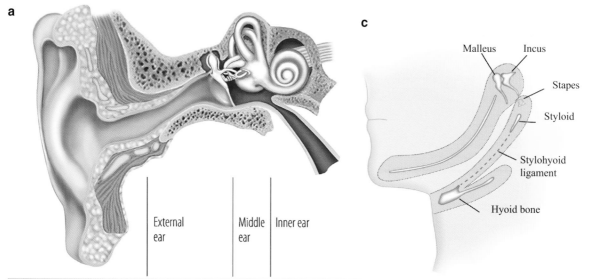

External
ear

Middle
ear

Inner ear

c

Malleus   Incus

Stapes

Styloid

Stylohyoid
ligament

Hyoid bone

b

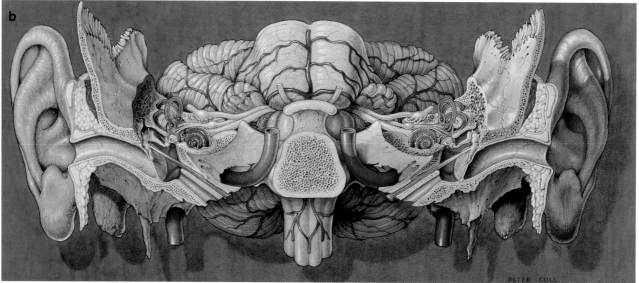

PETER CULL

Fig. 1.1.1 (**a**) The ear is divided into three compartments: external, middle, and inner. The pinna is composed of cartilage covered by skin. The shape of the cartilage is very important, since it gives the shape of the auricle. Any necrosis of the cartilage may lead to cosmetic deformity. The external auditory canal measures approximately 2.5 cm. The outer one-third is cartilaginous and the inner two-thirds is bony. There is a narrowing at the bone–cartilage junction which causes foreign bodies to get stuck in this area. The skin of the bony part is very thin lying on the periosteum and does not contain glands, hair follicles, and any adnexal structures. There are two or three fissures in the cartilaginous external auditory canal which are called "Santorini fissures." These fissures provide a potential route for the spread of infection from the external ear to the parotid area or infratemporal fossa and also of tumors from the parotid area to the external ear. The eustachian tube connects the middle ear to the nasopharynx. The posterior one-third of the adult eustachian tube is bony and lies within the petrous portion of the temporal bone. The anterior two-thirds is cartilaginous. In adults the tube lies at an angle of 45° in relation to the horizontal plane, whereas this inclination is only 10° in infants. The tube is longer in the adult than in the infant and young child. (**b**) Illustration showing the organs of hearing and the cerebellum. Sound waves are channeled by the pinna (visible part of the ear) into the auditory canal (*pink*) toward the eardrum. The eardrum transmits the vibrations to three tiny bones – the malleus, incus, and stapes – in the middle ear. The stapes passes the vibrations to the inner ear structures (*purple*), the semicircular canals and the cochlea (*spiral*). Auditory sensations are picked up by the cochlear nerve (*yellow*) and transmitted to the medulla (brainstem), the thalamus, and ultimately the cerebral cortex (visual photos). (**c**) The external and middle ear develop from the branchial apparatus. The middle ear cavity is derived from the endodermal first branchial cleft. The inner ear develops from the otic placode. The first arch, or Meckel's cartilage, contributes to the malleus and the incus. The tensor tympani muscle derives from the first branchial arch and is innervated by the nerve of the first branchial arch, which is mandibular branch of the trigeminal nerve. The second branchial arch, or Reichert's cartilage, contributes to the suprastructure of the stapes. The stapes muscle is innervated by a facial nerve, which is the nerve of the second branchial arch. The chorda tympani nerve, a branch of the facial nerve (second arch nerve), joins the first arch nerve to the mandibular lingual nerve. The footplate of the stapes is derived from the otic capsule. Thus, a congenital abnormality can occur in one part while the other parts may develop normally

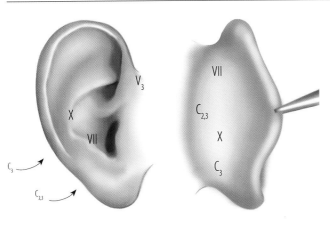

Fig. 1.1.2 The innervation of the auricle is by the greater auricular nerve (C3), the lesser occipital nerve (C2, 3), the auriculotemporal nerve (V3), and sensorial branches of the VII and X cranial nerves

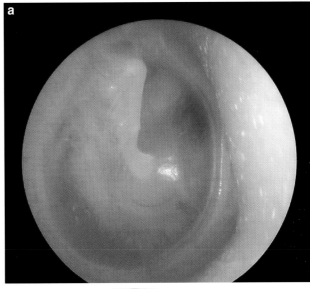

a

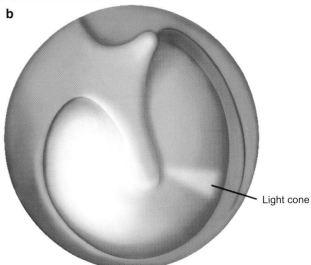

b

Light cone

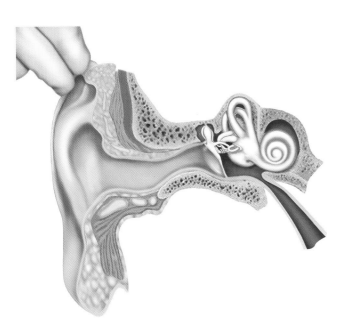

Fig. 1.1.3 The external auditory canal is not straight. To see the tympanic membrane, the ear canal should be straightened by pulling the auricle posteriorly and superiorly in adults (but inferiorly in infants)

Fig. 1.1.4 (a, b) The tympanic membrane is elliptical and slightly conical in shape. The apex of this cone, the umbo, marks the inferior part of the manubrium. The diameter of the tympanic membrane measures approximately 9 mm (9–10 vertical; 8–9 horizontal). The surface area is 85–90 mm^2. The tympanic membrane is composed of three layers: an outer epidermal layer, an inner mucosal layer, and a middle fibrous layer. The area above the short process of the malleus is known as pars flaccida and the area below as pars tensa. The pars flaccida does not have a middle fibrous layer, therefore it is flaccid. The pars tensa thickens peripherally forming the tympanic annulus. The tympanic annulus does not exist superiorly around the pars flaccida. There is a light triangle in the anterior–inferior quadrant of the tympanic membrane. The position of this triangle changes superiorly and becomes shorter when the tympanic membrane is retracted

Fig. 1.1.5 False-color scanning electron micrograph (SEM) of the three smallest bones in the human body responsible for conduction of sound waves in the middle ear. At the *top left* is the malleus (hammer), which strikes the incus (anvil – *right* of malleus); the incus is joined to the stapes (stirrups), which conducts sound toward the inner ear. Sound waves enter the ear through the external auditory meatus and cause the eardrum to vibrate. Vibrations from the eardrum are passed to the malleus and then the stapes via the incus. The stapes transmits the vibrations to the fluid-filled cochlea of the inner ear where the vibrations are converted to nerve impulses. Lever effect: the manubrium mallei is 1.3 times longer than the long process of the incus. This difference in the lengths of the manubrium mallei and long process of the incus contributes a lever factor of 1.3 to increase the intensity of the sound (visual photos)

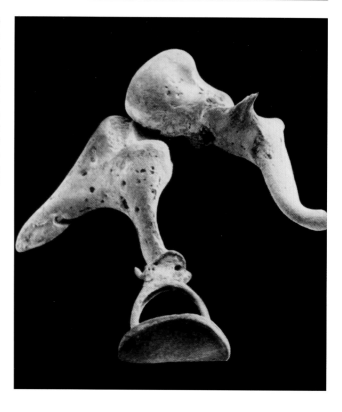

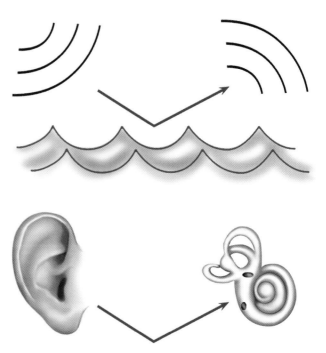

Fig. 1.1.6 Due to the differences in the physical properties of air and water, sound vibrations in the air are largely reflected away from the surface of water (99.9% of the energy of air-borne sound is reflected away), with only 0.1% entering the water. Although the surface area of the tympanic membrane is 85–90 mm², the effective vibrating area of the tympanic membrane is 55 mm². The surface area of the footplate is 3.2 mm². The ratio of the surface areas of the tympanic membrane and the footplate is $55/3.2 = 17.1$. This represents the hydraulic ratio of the tympanic membrane and stapes footplate, producing an increase force at the oval window of 17 times for the human ear, since the sound pressure level is equal to the force divided by the surface area ($P = F/a$). The final transformer ratio of the human tympanic membrane and ossicular chain is the product of the lever ratio of 1.3 times the hydraulic ratio of 17, which equals 22. This gain compensates the loss due to the air–bone difference

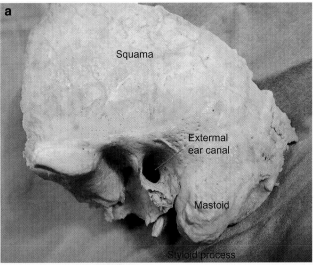

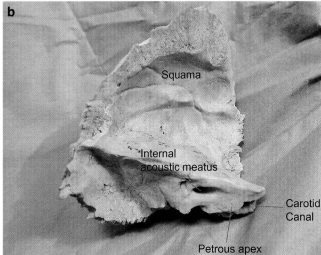

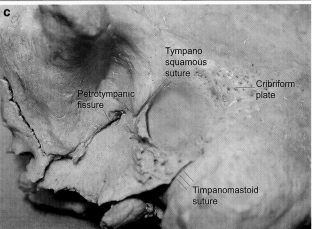

Fig. 1.1.7 (a–c) The temporal bone contains the ear. It has five parts: the bony external ear canal, the styloid process, the squamous portion, the petrous portion, and the mastoid process. There are suture lines between these various portions such as the petrotympanic fis-sure, petrosquamous suture, tympanosquamous suture, tympano-mastoid suture etc. The mastoid process is not present at birth, which makes the facial nerve very superficial

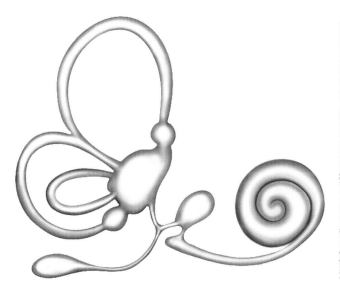

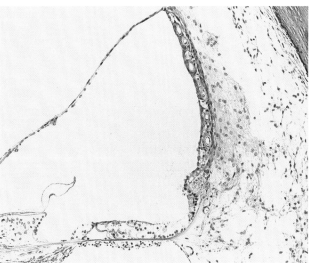

Fig. 1.1.8 The inner ear comprises the cochlea and the labyrinth. The labyrinth consists of three semicircular canals (superior, posterior, and lateral) and two otolithic organs (utricle and saccule). The utricu-lar duct and the saccular duct join to form the endolymphatic duct

Fig. 1.1.9 The cochlea has three fluid-filled compartments: the scala tympani, the scala vestibuli, and the scala media, which contains the organ of Corti (courtesy of Paparella, Paparella otopathology lab director)

Fig. 1.1.10 Inner ear organ of Corti. Color SEM of a section through the human inner ear, showing the organ of Corti (spiral organ). At the *top right* can be seen four rows of hair cells, supported by pillar-like Dieter cells. Each hair cell contains up to 100 individual hairs. The hairs translate mechanical movement caused by their displacement by sound waves into electrical impulses, which are transmitted to the brain via the cochlear nerve (visual photos)

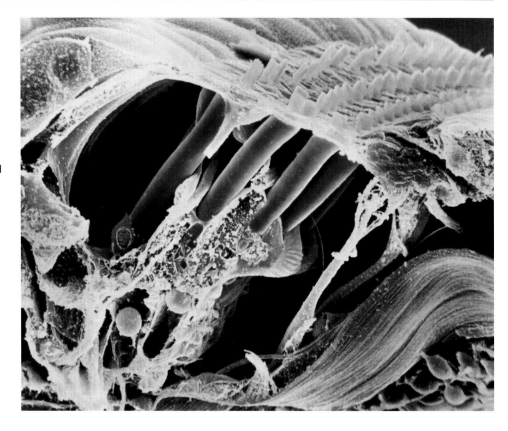

Fig. 1.1.11 Sensory hair cells in the ear. Color SEM of hair cells in the cochlea, the inner ear's auditory sense organ. The crescent-shaped areas across the center are numerous *stereocilia*, and are located on top of supporting hair cells. Sound waves entering the inner ear displace the fluid that surrounds the stereocilia, causing them to bend. This triggers a response in the hair cells, which release neurotransmitter chemicals that generate nerve impulses. The nerve impulses travel to the brain along the auditory nerve. This process can transmit information about the loudness and pitch of a sound. Magnification: ×2,000 when printed 10 cm wide (visual photos)

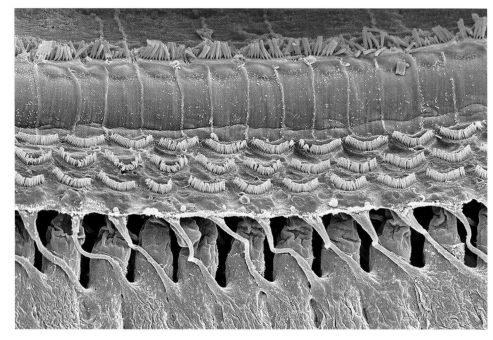

Fig. 1.1.12 Balancing stone from inner ear. Color SEM of crystals of calcium carbonate on the surface of an otolith. An otolith or *otoconium* is a calcified stone that is found in the otolith organs of the inner ear. They are attached to sensory hairs, and, when the head tilts, the movement of the stones causes nerve impulses that form the basis of the sense of balance. In humans, otoconia can range in size from 3 to 30 μm (millionths of a meter) across (visual photos)

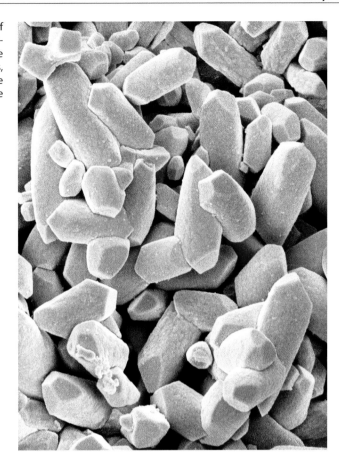

Table 1.1.1 Differences between anatomy of the eustachian tube (ET) in infants and adults

Anatomic features of the ET	Infants	Adults
Length of tube	Shorter	Longer
Lumen	Smaller	Wider
Angle of tube to horizontal plane	10°	45°
Mucosal folds	Greater	Lesser

1.2

ENT Examination

Tuning Fork Tests

Weber Test

Tuning fork tests are generally performed with a 512-Hz fork. The vibrating fork is placed on the patient's forehead. Sound lateralized to the poor hearing ear indicates a conductive hearing loss. Sound lateralized to the better hearing ear suggests a sensorineural hearing loss in the opposite ear.

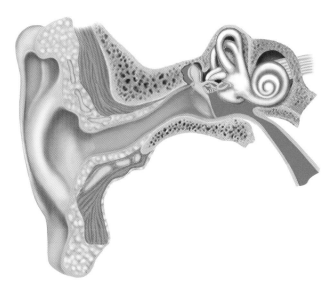

Fig. 1.2.1 Pathologies in the external and middle ear cause conductive hearing loss

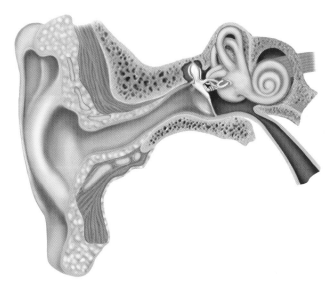

Fig. 1.2.2 Pathologies in the inner ear and the hearing nerve cause sensorineural hearing loss

Rinne Test

The vibrating fork is placed first on the mastoid bone. When the patient no longer hears, the tuning fork is brought 1 cm away from the external meatus. The result is expressed as "Rinne positive" when sound is heard longer by air, and "Rinne negative" when sound is heard longer by bone. Normally the sound of the fork is perceived louder when placed in front of the ear canal (Rinne positive).

False Rinne

When the fork is placed on the bone, the vibrations are conducted by bones of the skull to both cochleas. A patient with a total loss of hearing in one ear can hear the sound in the better ear by bone cross-conduction if the fork is placed on the mastoid bone of the diseased ear. The patient does not hear when the fork is brought in front of the external meatus after sound is no longer heard by mastoid bone conduction. The result is reported as a negative Rinne indicating the presence of conductive hearing loss, when in fact a false-negative Rinne has occurred.

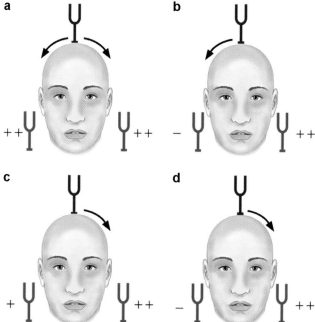

Fig. 1.2.3 Tuning fork tests. (**a**) Normal hearing: Weber test, the sound heard by both ears is equal, no lateralization; Rinne test bilateral +. (**b**) Conductive hearing loss in the right ear: Weber test, the sound is lateralized to the right ear; Rinne test is negative on the right ear, positive in the left ear. (**c**) Sensorineural hearing loss in the right ear: Weber test, the sound is lateralized to the left ear. Rinne test is positive in both ears; however, the duration is shorter in the right ear. (**d**) Total hearing loss in the right ear: Weber test, the sound is lateralized to the left. Rinne is positive in the left ear and negative in the right ear

EAR

NOSE

THROAT AND NECK

Table 1.2.1 Tuning fork tests and type of hearing loss

Rinne (diseased ear)	Weber	Type of hearing loss
Positive	Not lateralized	Normal hearing
Positive	Lateralized to the better ear	Sensorineural hearing loss
Negative	Lateralized to the diseased ear	Conductive hearing loss
Negative	Lateralized to the better ear	Total sensorineural hearing loss

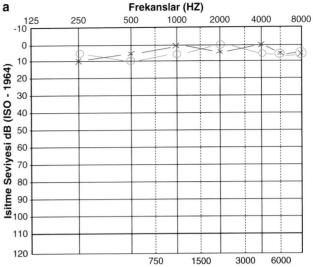

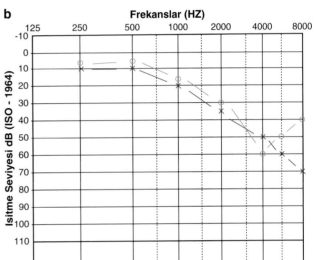

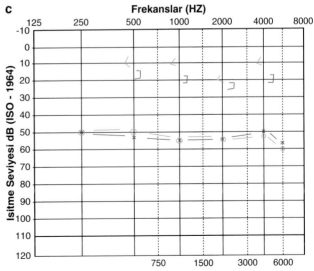

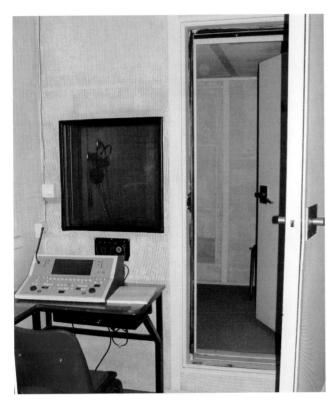

Fig. 1.2.4 Soundproof hearing test rooms

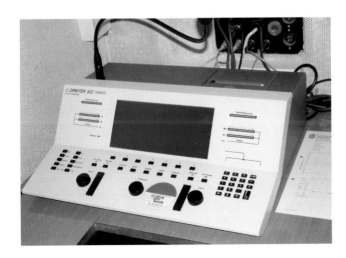

Fig. 1.2.6 Audiograms. (**a**) Normal hearing curve, (**b**) hearing loss due to acoustic trauma, (**c**) conductive-type hearing loss due to otosclerosis

Fig. 1.2.5 Audiometer to test hearing

Tympanometry

Tympanometry is an indirect measure of the mobility (compliance) of the tympanic membrane and ossicular chain under different pressures. The mobility of the tympanic membrane is greatest when the pressure on both sides of the tympanic membrane is equal. Compliance is reduced as air pressure is increased or decreased from normal. High acoustic energy is applied in the ear canal, some of this energy is absorbed and the remainder is reflected back and received by the probe. When the mobility is decreased, the energy is reflected more than the normal. In ears filled with fluid, tympanic membrane thickening, or ossicular chain stiffening, the reflected energy is greater than in normal ears.

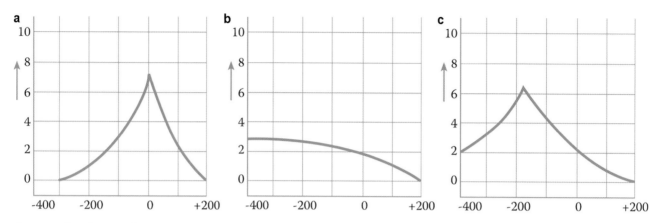

Fig. 1.2.7 Classification of tympanograms. **(a)** Type A: The curve peaks at 0 mm H$_2$O, indicating no pressure difference exists between the middle ear and the external environment. (If the peak of the curve is lower than the normal type A curve, stiffening of the ossicular chain is often associated. If the peak of the curve is very high, it suggests ossicular discontinuity). **(b)** Type B: The tympanogram is relatively flat or dome shaped. This shows little change in the reflective quality of the tympano-ossicular system as air pressures change in the external canal. This type of tympanogram is generally associated with middle ear fluid. **(c)** Type C: The peak of the curve occurs with higher negative pressures (maximum compliance is reached at negative pressures, meaning the pressure in the middle ear is negative). This curve indicates eustachian tube dysfunction

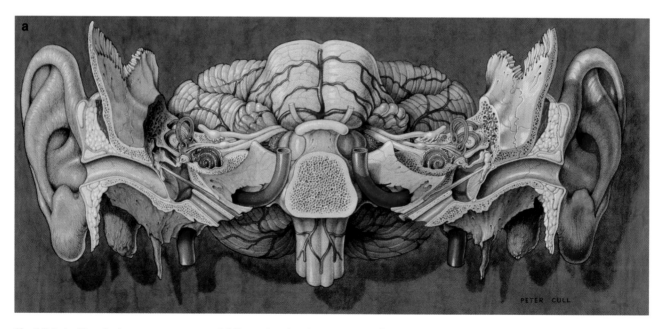

Fig. 1.2.8 Auditory brain stem response test. **(a)** Illustration showing the organs of hearing and the cerebellum. Sound waves are channeled by the pinna (visible part of the ear) into the auditory canal (*pink*) toward the eardrum. The eardrum transmits the vibrations to three tiny bones, the malleus, incus, and stapes, in the middle ear. The stapes passes the vibrations to the inner ear structures (*purple*), the semicircular canals and the cochlea (*spiral*). Auditory sensations are picked up by the cochlear nerve (*yellow*) and transmitted to the medulla (brain stem), the thalamus, and ultimately the cerebral cortex (visual photos). **(b)** The source of potentials. **(c)** Normal auditory brain stem response with six waves from five different anatomic sites

b

c

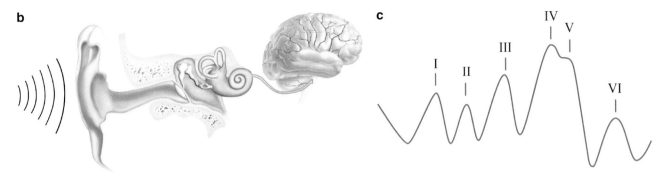

Fig. 1.2.8 (Continued)

Table 1.2.2 The source of the potentials (Fig. 1.2.8 a, b, c)

Anatomic localization	Wave
Cochlea, eighth nerve	I and II
Cochlear nucleus	III
Olivary complex	IV
Lateral lemniscus	V
Inferior colliculus	VI

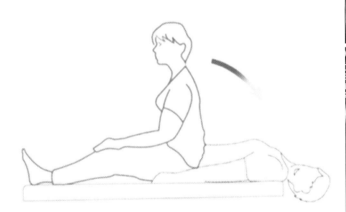

Fig. 1.2.9 Dix Hallpike maneuver for benign positional vertigo. Bringing the head to the head-hanging position may cause vertigo and nystagmus

Table 1.2.3 Differential diagnosis in positional vertigo

	Peripheral	Central
Latent period	+	−
Adaptation[a]	+	−
Fatigue[a]	+	−

[a]Vertigo adapts by holding the patient's head in the same position; vertigo fatigues on repeated positioning.

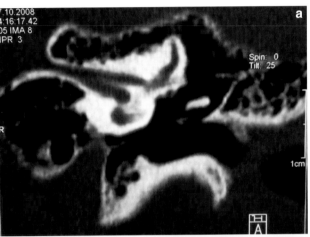

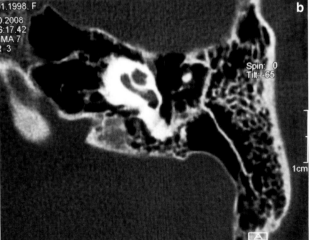

Fig. 1.2.10 (**a, b**) Temporal bone CT scans. External auditory meatus, middle ear cavity, attic, mastoid aircells, cochlea, semicircular canals, and internal acoustic canal (and falciform crest in the internal acoustic canal) can be seen

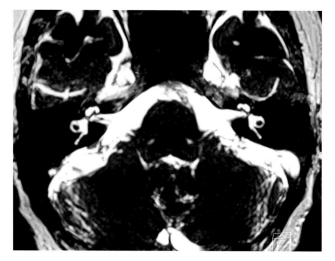

Fig. 1.2.11 Axial temporal MR image of the cochlea. Semicircular canals and cochlear and vestibular nerves can be identified

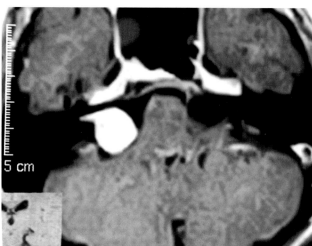

Fig. 1.2.12 Axial temporal MR shows acoustic neuroma in the left cerebellopontine angle

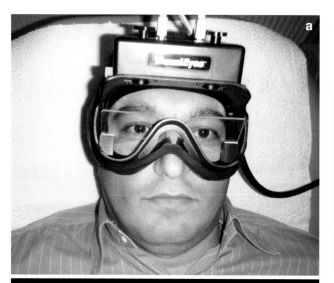

Fig. 1.2.13 (**a**, **b**) Electrovideonystagmography to record the eye movements and to analyze the nystagmus

Table 1.2.4 Causes of conductive hearing loss

Cerumen
Congenital ear atresia
Foreign body in the external ear canal
Hemotympanum
Chronic otitis media
Tympanic membrane perforation
Ossicular chain disruption
Temporal bone fractures, longitudinal
Benign tumors of the middle ear
Malignant tumors of the middle ear
Other

Table 1.2.5 Causes of sensorineural hearing loss

Presbyacusis
Noise-induced hearing loss
Ototoxicity
Endolymphatic hydrops
Acoustic neuroma
Labyrinthitis
Transverse temporal bone fracture
Enlarged vestibular aqueduct syndrome
Congenital inner ear abnormalities
Other

Vestibular tests should not be performed if the patient is taking vestibular suppressants or alcohol.

Electronystagmography (ENG) analyzes the eye movements. Eye movements that are tested include saccade, pursuit, and gaze. Saccade is a rapid eye movement made to bring the target onto the fovea. Pursuit is following a moving object. Gaze is fixation of the eyes on a target 20–30° bilaterally for at least 30 s. ENG recordings are also made with positional tests, optokinetic tests, and caloric tests.

All abnormalities in the oculomotor tests, such as in saccades, tracking, and gaze, indicate CNS disease. Failure of fixation suppression during caloric tests shows CNS disease.

Caloric test: Each ear is irrigated with water at 30 and 44°. Air may also be used for this purpose. The caloric stimulus causes nystagmus. Nystagmus is classified according to the direction of the fast phase. Cold stimulus causes nystagmus to the opposite side and warm stimulus causes nystagmus to the same side. The caloric test only tests the horizontal semicircular canals. More than 20% difference between the two ears is interpreted as weakness or canal paresis on that side.

Table 1.2.6 Electronystagmography abnormalities

Test with abnormality	Location of lesion
Saccade test	CNS
Gaze test	
Spontaneous nystagmus suppressed by visual fixation	Peripheral
Spontaneous nystagmus not suppressed by visual fixation	CNS
Unilateral or bilateral gaze nystagmus	CNS
Periodic alternating nystagmus	CNS
Rebound nystagmus	CNS
Upbeating or downbeating nystagmus	CNS
Tracking test	CNS
Optokinetic test	CNS

Table 1.2.7 Caloric test abnormalities

Unilateral or bilateral weakness	Peripheral
Directional preponderance	Peripheral or CNS
Failure of fixation suppression	CNS
Caloric inversion or perversion	CNS

1.3

The Pinna

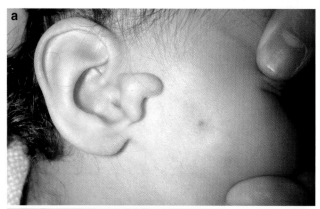

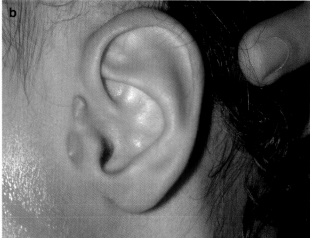

Fig. 1.3.1 (a) Preauricular skin tags are generally unilateral. They can be removed before school age if they cause cosmetic deformities. **(b)** Cartilage remnants in front of the tragus

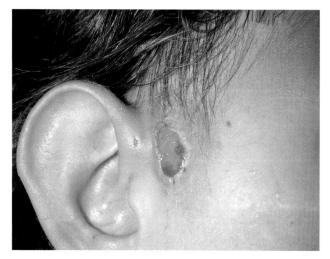

Fig. 1.3.2 Preauricular fistulas are due to fusion abnormalities during embryogenic development of the auricle. Seventy-five percent of cases are unilateral. If the orifice of the fistula is narrow, the debris may occlude the orifice and cause secondary infection. The whole sinus tract should be removed surgically

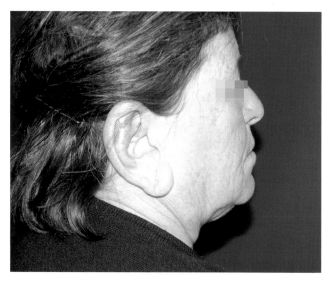

Fig. 1.3.3 Macrotia is a large pinna

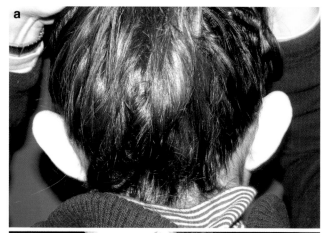

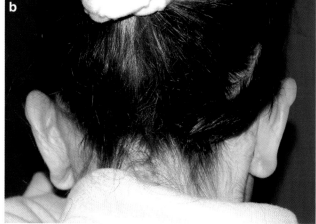

Fig. 1.3.4 Prominent ear. **(a)** Posterior view before the operation and **(b)** 3 months after the operation. In prominent ears, the fold of the antihelix is either absent or poorly formed and the angle between the posterior surface of the conchal cartilage and the cranium is over 300°. There is an autosomal dominant inheritance. It is also referred to as bat ears or lop ears. Prominent ears should be corrected before school age, between 4 and 6 years

Fig. 1.3.5 Abnormalities of the auricle range from minor abnormalities that require no treatment to total absence of the pinna. Since the embryological development of the pinna is completely different from the middle and inner ear, it is not generally associated with middle and inner ear abnormalities. However, atresia of the external ear canal may accompany microtia. (**a**, **b**) In type I microtia deformity, the deformity is only limited to the helix and antihelix and it is a minimal deformity. (**c**, **d**) In type II there is severe deformity, although the remnant of the pinna is present. (**e**, **f**) In type III deformity there is no pinna. Generally the external ear canal is completely atresic. In some patients the lobule may be present. The optimum age for surgery is around 5 years, until the other auricle reaches its adult size and the costal cartilage development is sufficient to be used in reconstruction. It is also important to operate on children before school age

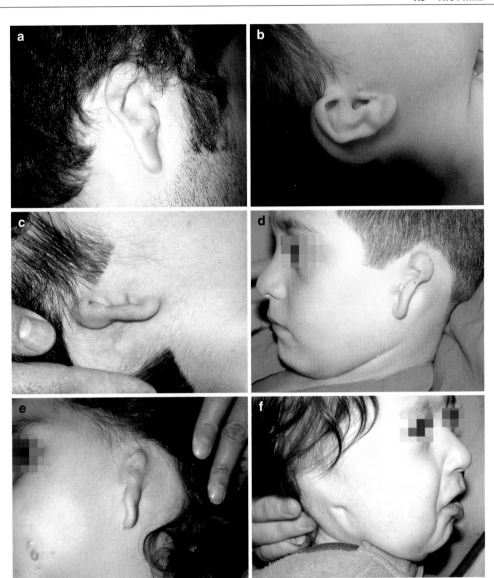

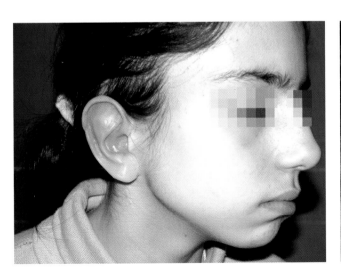

Fig. 1.3.6 In the complete absence of the auricle, an auricular implant may give a natural appearance

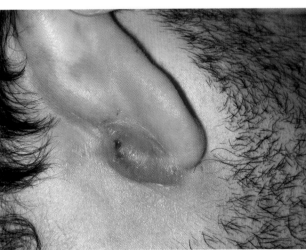

Fig. 1.3.7 Sebaceous cyst in the postauricular sulcus. Complete removal is necessary to prevent recurrences

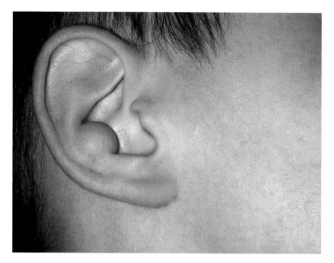

Fig. 1.3.8 A benign mass located in the anteroinferior part of the helix

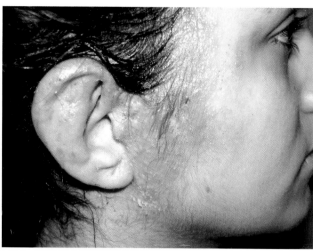

Fig. 1.3.10 A burn in the preauricular skin and pinna due to cleaning with pure antiseptic agent (Courtesy of TESAV)

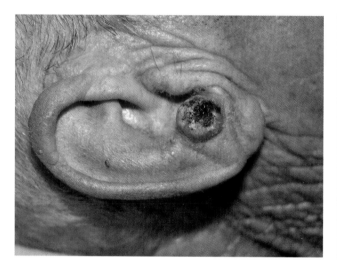

Fig. 1.3.9 Malignant tumor in the auricle

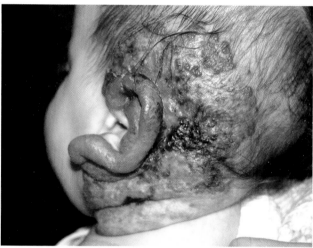

Fig. 1.3.11 Hemangioma at the auricle. These tumors may regress spontaneously. Steroid treatment for young patients under 1 year of age may be useful (Courtesy of TESAV)

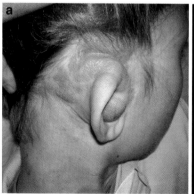
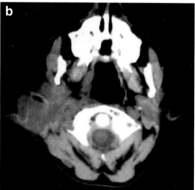
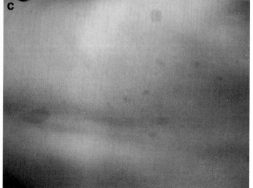

Fig. 1.3.12 (a) Neurofibromas of the pinna. (b) Axial CT image shows massive involvement of the deep tissue planes. (c) Cafe-au-lait spots, which are characteristic of NF1, are also frequently seen in patients with NF2. Neurofibromas may be solitary or may occur as part of neurofibromatosis in patients with Recklinghausen's disease. Solitary neurofibromas should be excised if they cause functional or cosmetic problems. Since these tumors have malignant potential, any change in the behavior of the tumor such as sudden increase in size, pain etc. should warn the surgeon about the possibility of malignancy. Extensive surgery is required for massive tumours. Conservative management is the best option

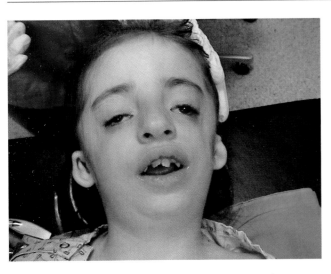

Fig. 1.3.13 Treacher Collins syndrome is a hereditary condition causing auricular deformities, abnormalities of the external ear, and hearing loss

1.4

External Ear Canal

Table 1.4.1 Differential diagnosis between acute mastoiditis and furunculosis

	Acute mastoiditis	Furunculosis
History of acute otitis media	+	–
Hearing loss	+	– (only if external ear canal is occluded)
Tympanic membrane	Hyperemic or bulging	Normal (if can be seen)
Pain on the mastoid area	+	–
Pain with manipulation of pinna or tragus	–	+
Postauricular sulcus	May be obliterated	Present
X–ray	Mastoids opaque	Mastoids normal

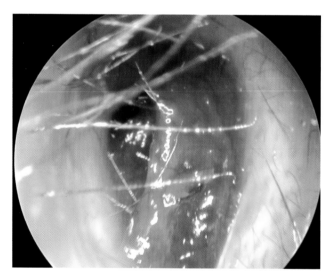

Fig. 1.4.1 If cerumen completely fills the external ear canal, it may cause conductive type hearing loss. Cerumen is the product of both sebaceous and apocrine glands which are located in the cartilaginous portion of the external ear canal. There are two basic types, "wet" and "dry." Caucasians have a greater than 80% probability of having wet, sticky, honey-colored ear wax. In the Mongoloid races the dry, scaly, rice-brand type is more common

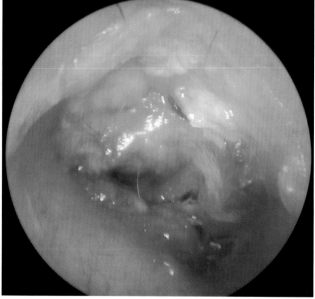

Fig. 1.4.2 Cerumen deep in the external ear canal preventing much of the tympanic membrane from being seen

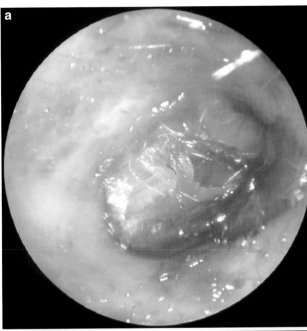

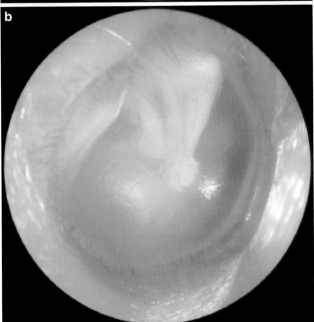

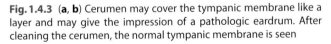

Fig. 1.4.3 (**a**, **b**) Cerumen may cover the tympanic membrane like a layer and may give the impression of a pathologic eardrum. After cleaning the cerumen, the normal tympanic membrane is seen

Fig. 1.4.5 (**a**) Removal of cerumen is done either by an ear curette or syringing. Adequate visualization and exposure is necessary to avoid trauma. If the cerumen is not hard enough, it may be removed with suction after being softened by ear drops. (**b**) Water irrigation is another method. After the ear canal has been straightened by pulling the pinna backward and upward, water at body temperature is administered in the posterosuperior direction. The water passes between the ear canal and the cerumen and pushes the cerumen outward. If the tympanic membrane is perforated, ear irrigation should not be done

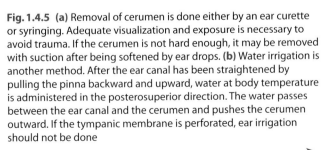

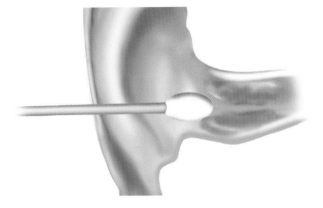

Fig. 1.4.4 In some people there is excessive cerumen production. The cerumen is generally occluded in the narrowest part of the external ear canal at its midportion. These patients need periodic cleaning. Use of cotton swabs can push the cerumen deeper in the ear canal, which occludes the ear canal completely and makes removal more difficult

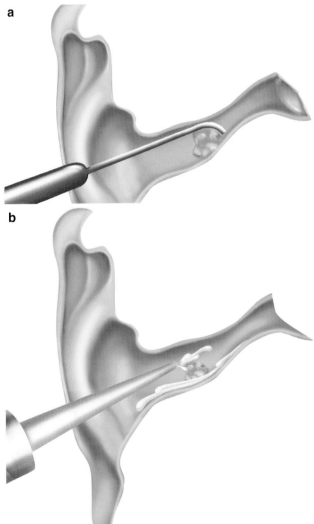

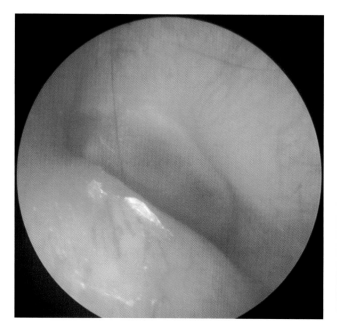

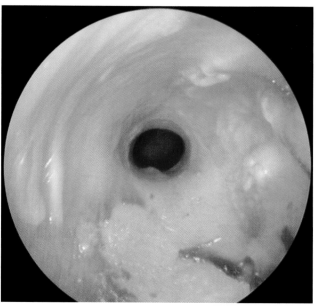

Fig. 1.4.6 Anterior wall of the external ear canal is prominent preventing the anterior part of the eardrum from being seen

Fig. 1.4.8 External auditory canal stenosis in a diabetic patient due to recurrent ear canal infections and trauma

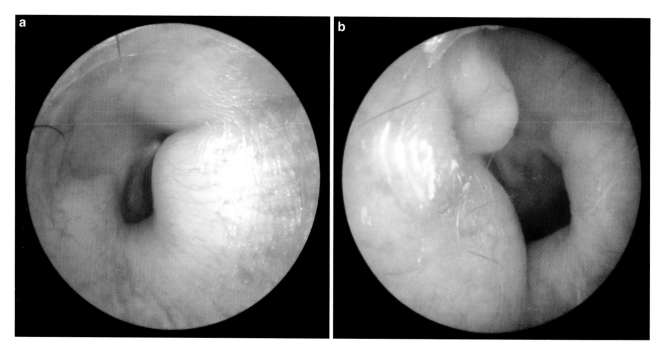

Fig. 1.4.7 (**a**, **b**) Exostoses may narrow the external ear canal and may cause debris and cerumen to collect behind them. They are generally seen in swimmers. They are bony, hard, and usually remain small and symptom free. They do not require any treatment unless they cause problems

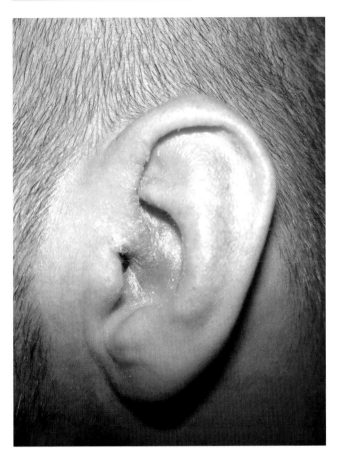

Fig. 1.4.9 Acute otitis externa. The ear canal is hyperemic and narrowed due to swelling. Manipulation of the auricle or tragus is painful

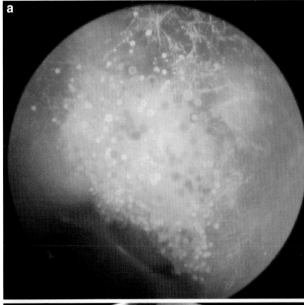

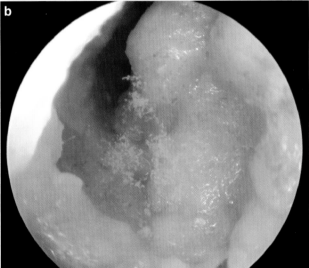

Fig. 1.4.11 (**a**, **b**) Otomycosis. Several fungi may cause infections in the external ear canal. The most common type is *Aspergillus* (*A. niger* or *A. flavus*). *Candida* may occasionally be the agent. Fungal hyphae may be seen in the external ear canal

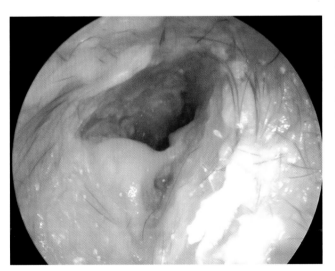

Fig. 1.4.10 Acute otitis externa. The ear canal is slightly narrowed due to swelling and is full of cerumen and purulent material

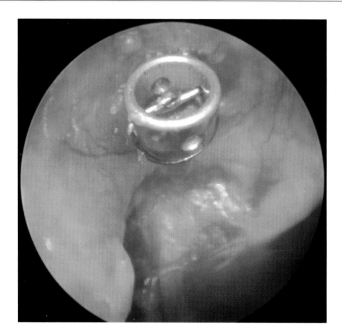

Fig. 1.4.12 Metal piston used in a stapedectomy was extruded into the external ear canal

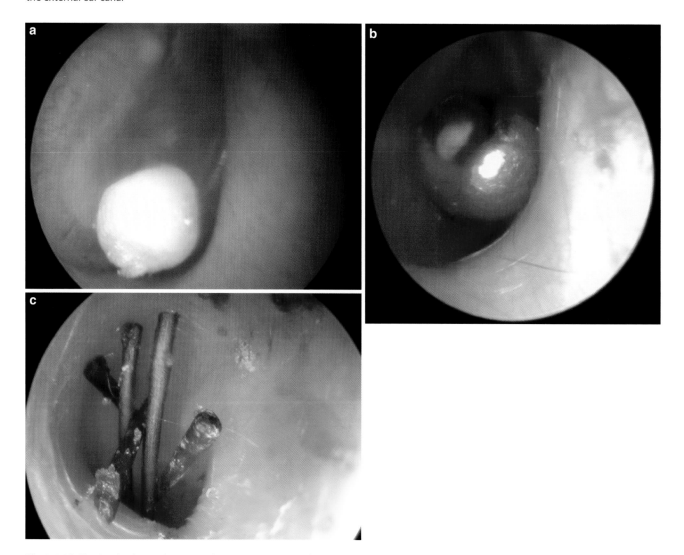

Fig. 1.4.13 Foreign bodies in the external ear canal. (**a**) Foam, (**b**) red bead, (**c**) pencil sticks used for scratching the external ear canal

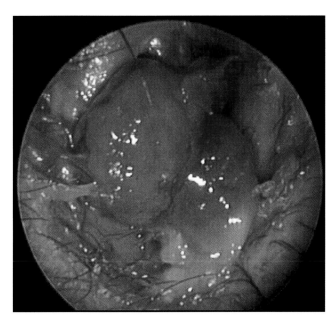

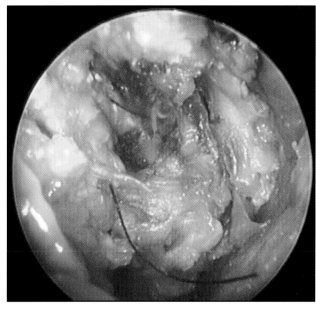

Fig. 1.4.14 Polyp extruding from the external auditory canal. It should be examined histologically

Fig. 1.4.15 Keratosis obturans. Desquamated epithelium accumulates and may form a large impacted mass in the meatus, causing erosion of the bony canal

1.5

Otitis Media with Effusion

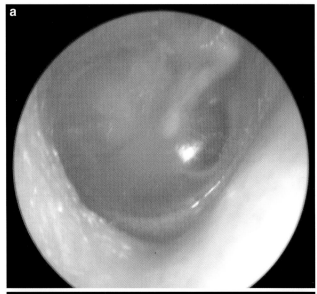

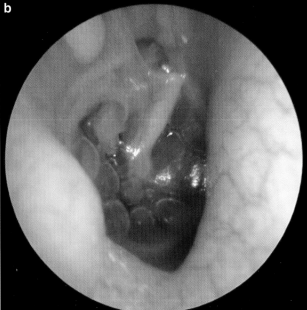

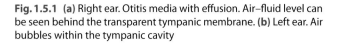

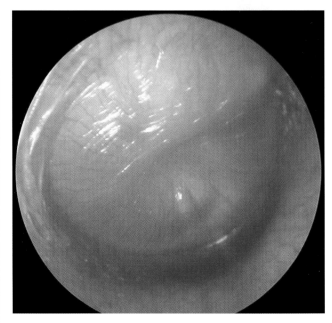

Fig. 1.5.2 Right ear. The tympanic membrane is vascularized and the transparency of the tympanic membrane is slightly diminished

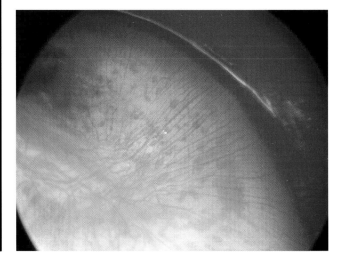

Fig. 1.5.1 **(a)** Right ear. Otitis media with effusion. Air–fluid level can be seen behind the transparent tympanic membrane. **(b)** Left ear. Air bubbles within the tympanic cavity

Fig. 1.5.3 Right ear: otitis media with effusion. In long-standing effusions the tympanic membrane has a dull or opaque appearance with vascularization on it

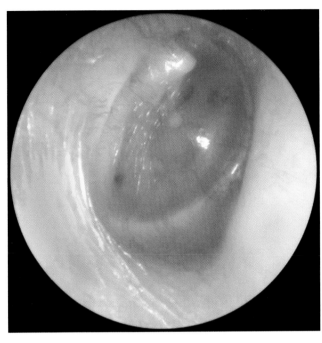

Fig. 1.5.4 Right ear. Otitis media with effusion. The tympanic membrane is opaque, has lost its transparency, is vascularized, and retracted. Please note that the light reflex is shorter and moved upward due to retraction of the tympanic membrane

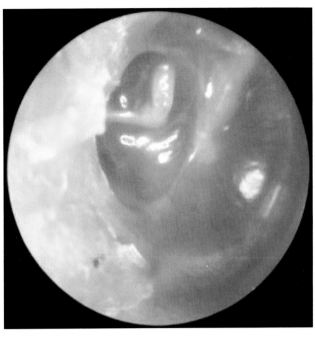

Fig. 1.5.6 Right ear. In long-standing effusions the retraction pockets most frequently develop in the posterosuperior part of the tympanic membrane. The retraction pocket just behind the malleus handle is seen and its apex can be identified. The pocket is clean containing no debris. The membrane lies on the incus and stapes. Behind the translucent thinned tympanic membrane, the incudostapedial joint and stapes tendon are clearly seen

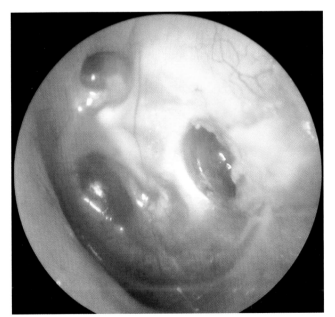

Fig. 1.5.5 Left ear. Otitis media with effusion. Retractions occur mostly in the weak parts of the tympanic membrane, such as the pseudomembranous parts or pars flaccida due to middle ear negative pressures

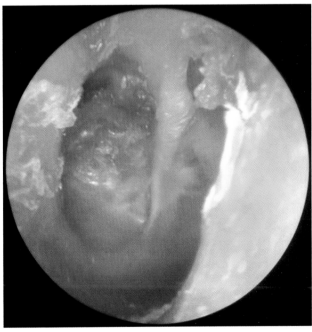

Fig. 1.5.7 Right ear. Retraction pocket with debris in it

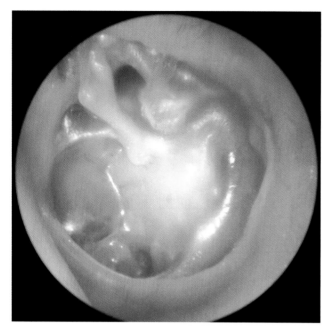

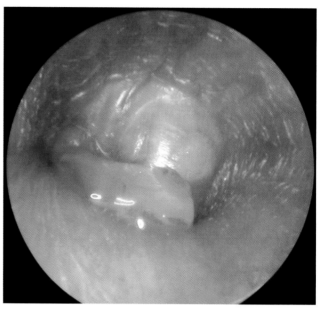

Fig. 1.5.10 Mucoid material in the external ear canal after myringotomy in otitis media with effusion

Fig. 1.5.8 Left ear. Adhesive otitis media. The tympanic membrane is thinned and lies on the promontorium. The short process of the malleus and malleus handle is more prominent due to retraction of the membrane. Fibrous annulus is clearly identified

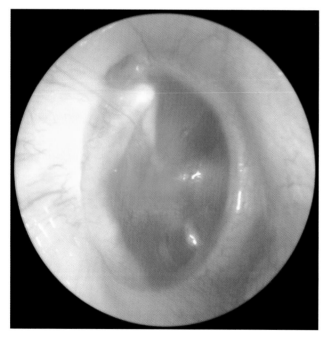

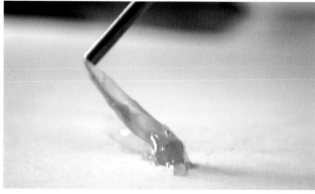

Fig. 1.5.11 Thick and sticky mucoid material obtained from the middle ear in a patient with otitis media with effusion

Fig. 1.5.9 Right ear. Otitis media with effusion due to nasopharyngeal carcinoma. Amber color and retraction of the tympanic membrane. A unilateral otitis media with effusion in adults always necessitates a detailed search for nasopharyngeal carcinoma

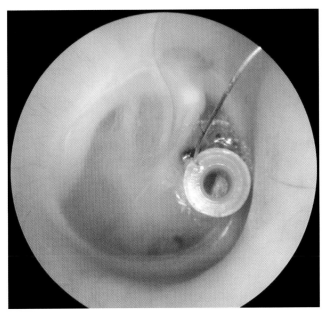

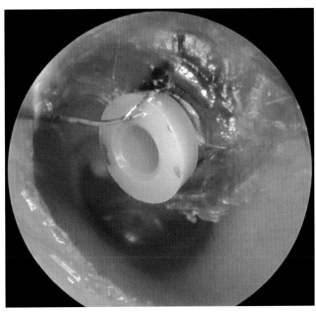

Fig. 1.5.12 Right ear. Sheppard grommet ventilation tube, which was inserted due to otitis media with effusion 6 months earlier. The tympanic membrane looks normal. The ventilation tubes ventilate the middle ear. The appearance of the drum returns to normal after a while. The tubes should stay in place for at least 6 months or more to have a normal middle ear physiology

Fig. 1.5.14 Sheppard grommet ventilation tube extrusion. A tube in the external ear canal with wax around it, 8 months after insertion. After extrusion, tympanosclerosis or membrane scarring may occur. A small tube causes less trauma but is extruded more rapidly

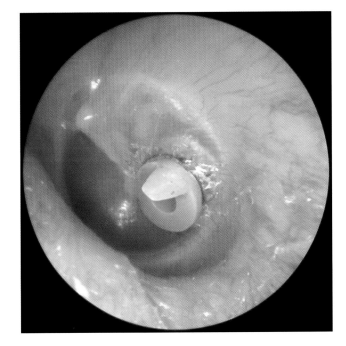

Fig. 1.5.13 Left ear. A 1.25-mm Paparella drain tube in the posterior inferior quadrant of the tympanic membrane. The tympanic membrane appears normal after 3 months of insertion of the ventilation tubes. Behind the transparent tympanic membrane the inner flanges of the tube can be seen. A myringotomy incision is generally made in the posterior inferior quadrant of the tympanic membrane. Some surgeons prefer to insert it in the anterosuperior quadrant to reduce the risk of early extrusion. Insertion of the ventilation tubes in the posterosuperior quadrant of the tympanic membrane should be avoided since it may damage the incudostapedial joint or long process of the incus

1.6

Acute Otitis Media

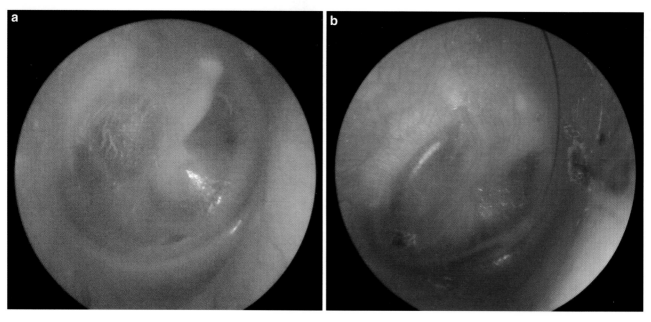

Fig. 1.6.1 **(a)** Normal tympanic membrane. The short process of the malleus and malleus handle is seen. The tympanic membrane is transparent, sometimes allowing the long process of the incus and promontorium to be seen. Note the light reflex in the anteroinferior quadrant of the membrane. **(b)** Eustachian tube dysfunction. Note the vascularization along the manubrium mallei

Fig. 1.6.2 Otitic barotrauma (hemotympanum). The tympanic membrane appears *blue* due to hemorrhagic fluid collected in the middle ear. It is due to an inability to ventilate the middle ear following an abnormal function of the eustachian tube. Otitic barotrauma is usually seen during descent in flight or during scuba diving. No treatment is needed. If there is associated upper respiratory tract infection or allergy, topical and systemic oral decongestants with antihistamines may help recovery. To prevent further episodes the patients are advised not to go scuba diving when their nose is obstructed because of the difficulty of inflating the eustachian tube. Frequent flyers and regular sufferers are advised to use prophylactic measures to prevent eustachian tube problems, such as topical nasal decongestants and chewing gum etc.

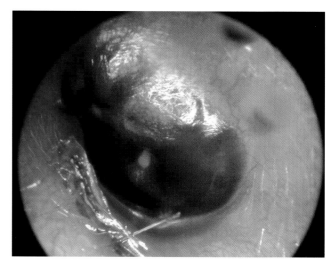

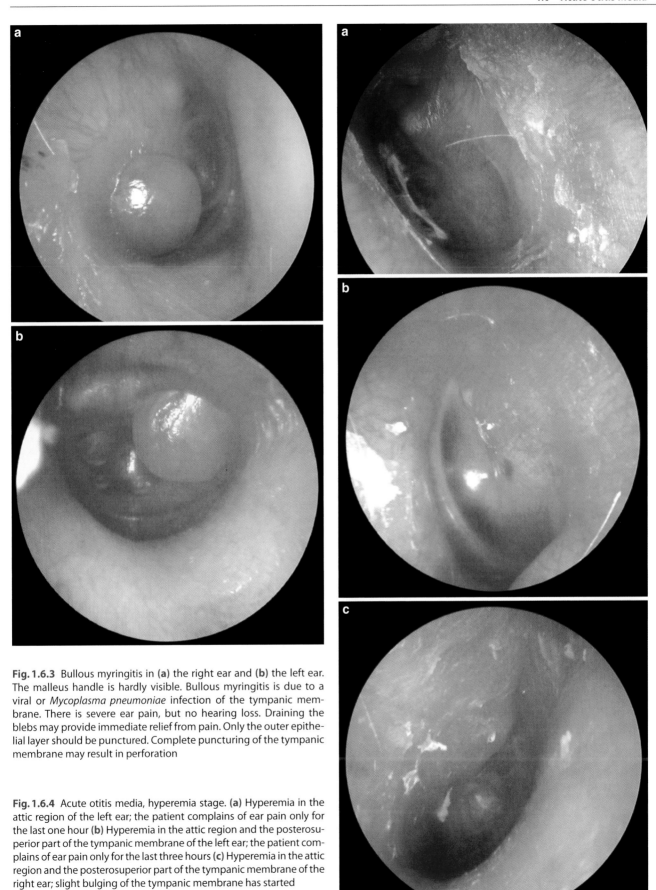

Fig. 1.6.3 Bullous myringitis in (**a**) the right ear and (**b**) the left ear. The malleus handle is hardly visible. Bullous myringitis is due to a viral or *Mycoplasma pneumoniae* infection of the tympanic membrane. There is severe ear pain, but no hearing loss. Draining the blebs may provide immediate relief from pain. Only the outer epithelial layer should be punctured. Complete puncturing of the tympanic membrane may result in perforation

Fig. 1.6.4 Acute otitis media, hyperemia stage. (**a**) Hyperemia in the attic region of the left ear; the patient complains of ear pain only for the last one hour (**b**) Hyperemia in the attic region and the posterosuperior part of the tympanic membrane of the left ear; the patient complains of ear pain only for the last three hours (**c**) Hyperemia in the attic region and the posterosuperior part of the tympanic membrane of the right ear; slight bulging of the tympanic membrane has started

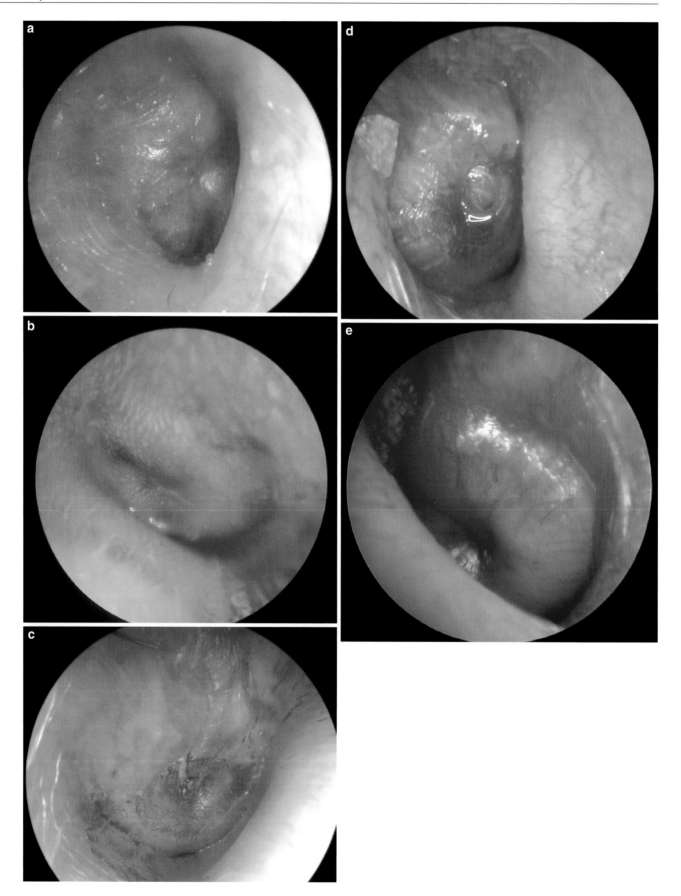

Fig. 1.6.5 Acute otitis media. Different phases of the exudative stage. (a) Bulging in the posterior half of the tympanic membrane (right ear). (b) Slight bulging of the tympanic membrane (left ear). (c) Due to bulging the malleus handle cannot be differentiated (right ear). (d) More severe bulging (right ear). (e) More severe bulging and opaque tympanic membrane (left ear). There is conductive-type hearing loss

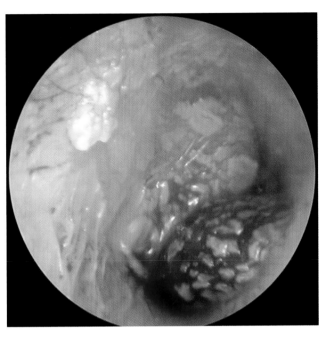

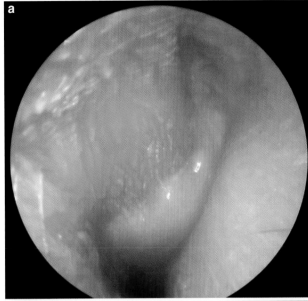

Fig. 1.6.6 Acute hemorrhagic otitis media in the right ear. Bulging of the tympanic membrane due to hemorrhagic purulent material in the middle ear

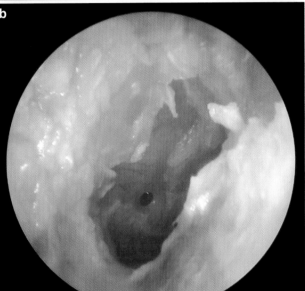

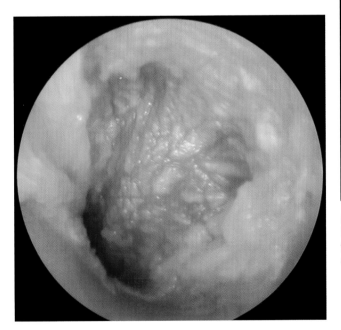

Fig. 1.6.8 Suppurative stage in acute otitis media (right ear). **(a)** Purulent material filling the external ear canal and preventing the drum from being seen. **(b)** The small perforations in the tympanic membrane are seen after cleaning the purulent material in the external ear

Fig. 1.6.7 Acute hemorrhagic otitis media in the right ear. There is severe bulging associated with severe ear pain. Due to extensive bulging, white-colored epithelium is seen on the tympanic membrane. The malleus cannot be identified

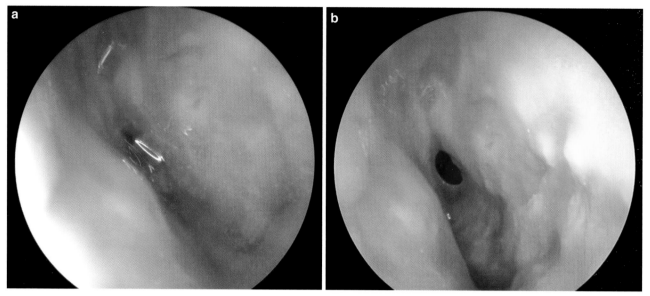

Fig. 1.6.9 Suppurative stage in acute otitis media (left ear). (**a**) Purulent material filling the external ear canal and preventing the drum from being seen. (**b**) The small perforations in the tympanic membrane are seen after cleaning the purulent material in the external ear. Note the perforation is located at the anterior superior quadrant. If drainage is not adequate, myringotomy at the lower quadrants may be necessary

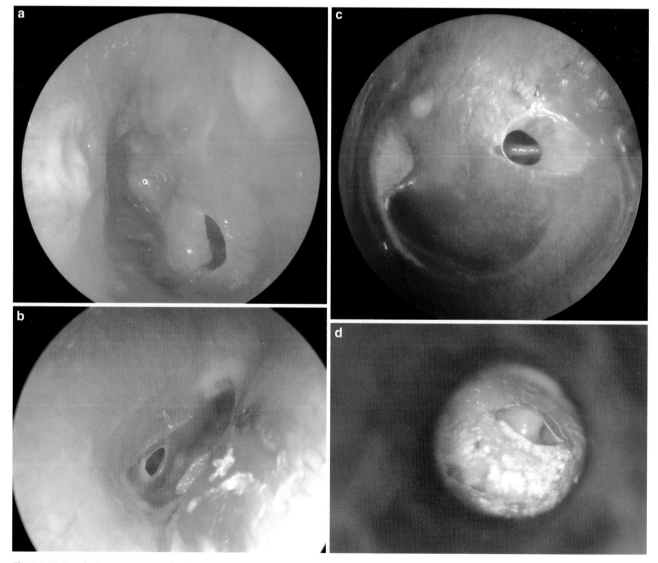

Fig. 1.6.10 Resolution stage. During healing small perforations are seen in different parts of the tympanic membrane. All these perforations close by themselves without any additional treatment. (**a**) Left ear; (**b**) right ear; (**c**) left ear, stapes muscle tendon is seen through the perforation; (**d**) left ear

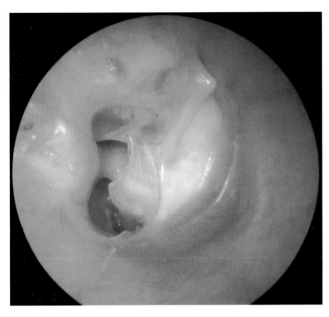

Fig. 1.6.11 The perforations of the tympanic membrane close by the epithelium coming from the edges of the perforation. Sometimes minor interventions may be needed if the perforation is big

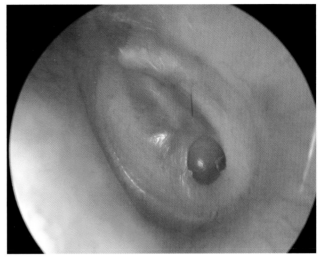

Fig. 1.6.13 The perforation closed by pseudomembrane formation

Table 1.6.1 Contributing factors for recurrent acute otitis media

Day care center
Smoking at home
Bottle feeding
No mother milk nutrition
Immune insufficiency
Cleft palate

Table 1.6.2 Pathogenesis of acute otitis media

Upper respiratory tract infection
Edema of the eustachian tube
Nasal obstruction
Positive pressure in the nasopharynx
Adenoid vegetation
Eustachian tube obstruction
Inhabit the pathogens

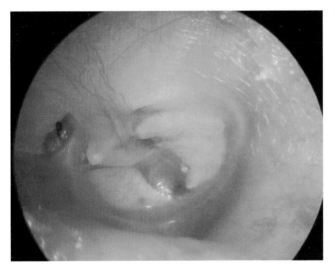

Fig. 1.6.12 White areas of tympanosclerosis. They do not cause any symptoms and any hearing loss. There is no need for treatment. Tympanosclerosis in the tympanic membrane generally follows the insertion of ventilation tubes. Previous otitis media may also cause tympanosclerosis in the tympanic membrane and ossicles. If tympanosclerosis reduces the mobility of the ossicles, conductive-type hearing loss may appear which is not so easy to treat

Table 1.6.3 Stages of acute otitis media

Hyperemia
Exudation
Suppuration
Coalescence
Complication
Resolution

1.7

Chronic Otitis Media

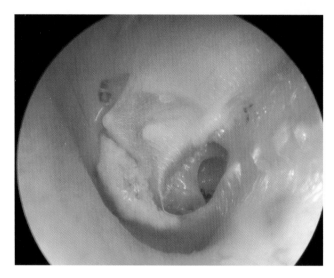

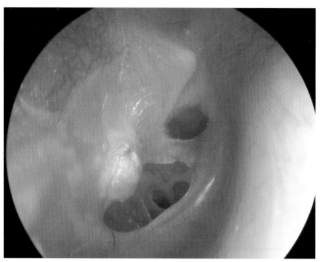

Fig. 1.7.1 Left ear. In the posteroinferior part of the tympanic membrane there is a central perforation. The epithelium goes into the middle ear from the anterior and inferior edges of the perforation. Anterior to the manubrium mallei the tympanic membrane is calcified. In the posterosuperior quadrant the tympanic membrane lies on the incus and stapes

Fig. 1.7.3 Right ear. Central perforation in the anteroinferior quadrant of the tympanic membrane. Pseudomembranous tympanic membrane in the anterosuperior quadrant. The middle ear mucosa and the tympanic membrane are tympanosclerotic. Just posteroinferior to the umbo, the tympanic membrane is thickened by fibrous tissue and embedded with calcium. Tympanosclerosis is the collection of collagen and calcium in the submucosal layer in the tympanic membrane or middle ear mucosa. It is a healing process of the body. Especially after ventilation tube insertion, white calcium deposits may be seen due to submucosal bleeding. Such tympanosclerotic plaques may be large enough to interfere with normal tympanic membrane function. In the middle ear mucosa it may cause fixation of the ossicles and may lead to conductive-type hearing loss

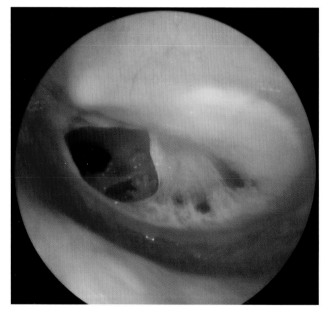

Fig. 1.7.2 Left ear. A central perforation in the anterosuperior quadrant of the tympanic membrane. Through the perforation the eustachian tube orifice and tympanosclerotic middle ear mucosa are seen. The tympanic membrane appears to be tympanosclerotic

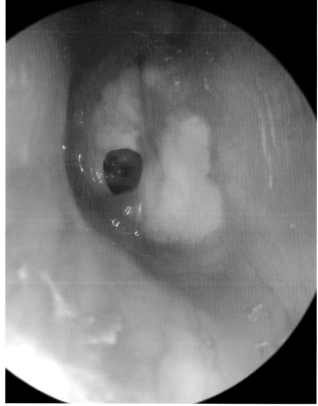

Fig. 1.7.4 Left ear. Anteroinferior central perforation. At the posteroinferior location of the perforation, polypoid granulation tissue is present; the middle ear mucosa is hyperemic and edematous. There are calcified plaques in the tympanic membrane

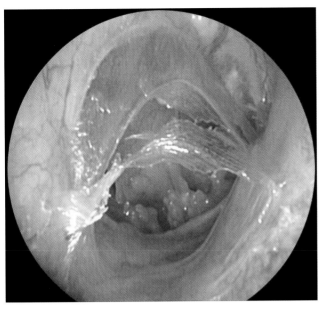

Fig. 1.7.5 Right ear. Central perforation with tympanosclerosis in the middle ear. The tympanic membrane tries to close the perforation and a pseudomembrane formation is seen

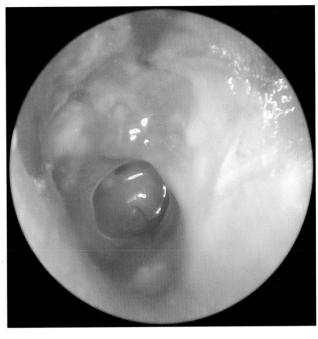

Fig. 1.7.7 Left ear. Acute infection in a patient with chronic otitis media. Purulent drainage in the external ear canal. There is a 3-mm central perforation in the tympanic membrane. Anterosuperior to the perforation there is polypoid tissue formation. The middle ear mucosa is edematous and hyperemic

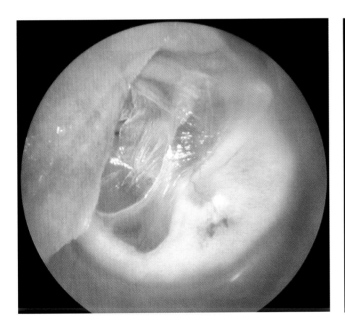

Fig. 1.7.6 Right ear. The anterior part is tympanosclerotic. The filter paper used to close the perforation is transported out onto the external ear canal and a replacement membrane closing the perforation is seen; however, there is a very small perforation still remaining between the filter paper and the pseudomembrane

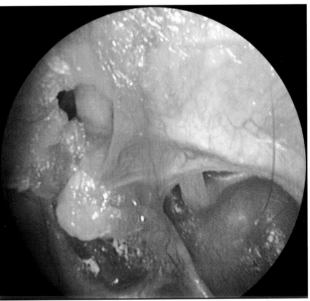

Fig. 1.7.8 Right ear. Short process of the malleus and malleus handle can be seen. Just above the short process, attic perforation is seen. Posterior to the malleus handle, the tympanic membrane is severely retracted and lies on the promontorium and incudostapedial joint. The long process of the incus, lenticular process, incudostapedial joint, and stapes tendon are seen behind the adhesive and thinned tympanic membrane

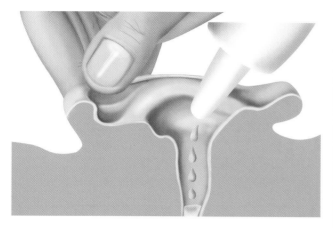

Fig. 1.7.9 Correct instillation of ear drops. First, any debris or discharge in the external ear canal is cleaned. The auricle is pulled upward and backward. Subsequently, five to six drops (or more if needed) are introduced into the ear canal (help may be needed). Tragal massage may help the drops go into the middle ear. The patient is kept in that position for 2–3 min. Cotton wool is placed in the ear canal and can be removed 10 min later

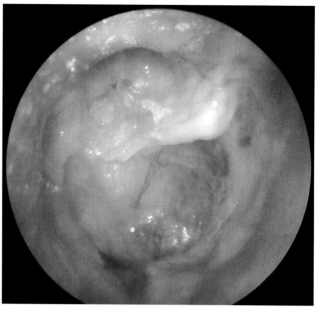

Fig. 1.7.11 Right ear. The tympanic membrane in the posterosuperior quadrant behind the malleus handle is retracted. The retraction pocket has cerumen and keratin debris and the apex of the retraction pocket cannot be identified

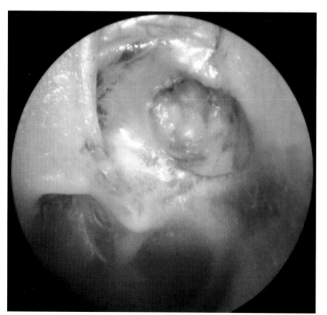

Fig. 1.7.10 Right ear. Attic perforation above the short process of the malleus after cleaning the epithelial debris

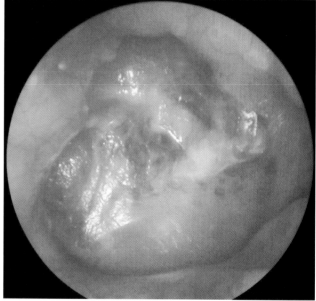

Fig. 1.7.12 Right ear. The tympanic membrane is retracted posterosuperiorly toward the antrum area. The bone over the retraction pocket is destroyed. The incus is eroded. The epithelium at the apex of the retraction pocket is seen. The chorda tympani nerve is visible behind the thinned retracted tympanic membrane

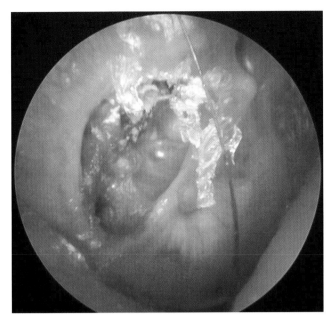

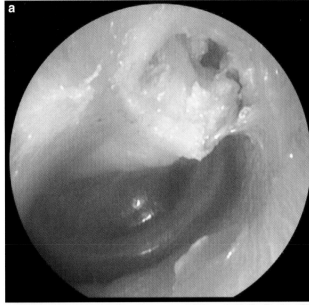

Fig. 1.7.13 Right ear. Behind the handle of the malleus, cerumen and keratin debris in the retraction pocket can be seen. The rest of the tympanic membrane is opaque and vascularized

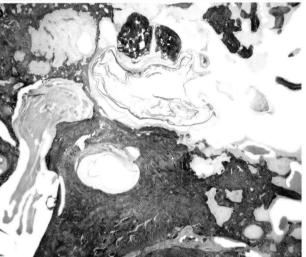

Fig. 1.7.15 (a) Right ear. Attic perforation and attic cholesteatoma above the short process of the malleus. (b) Histologic section of the temporal bone shows cholesteatoma in the attic (courtesy of Paparella, Paparella otopathology lab director)

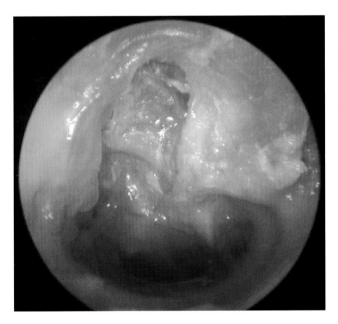

Fig. 1.7.14 Right ear. Cholesteatoma defect in the attic and antrum area. The cholesteatoma mass destroyed the bone at the attic region. The chorda tympani nerve is crossing the middle ear

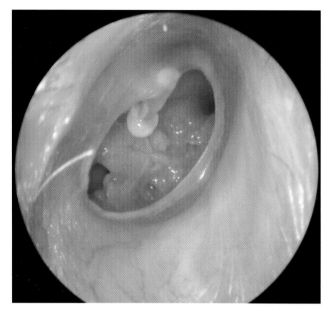

Fig. 1.7.16 Right ear. Subtotal perforation of the tympanic membrane. Short process of the malleus, malleus handle, umbo, and fibrous annulus are seen. In the anterosuperior part of the middle ear is the eustachian tube orifice and just above it facial nerve protuberance; in the posteroinferior part of the middle ear, round window niche is visible

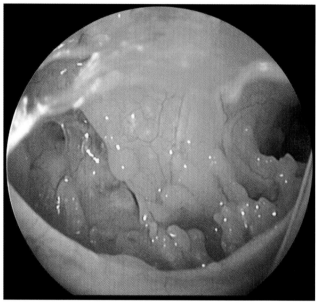

Fig. 1.7.18 Right ear. Nearly total tympanic membrane perforation. The middle ear mucosa is tympanosclerotic. In the anterosuperior part of the middle ear the eustachian tube orifice is seen

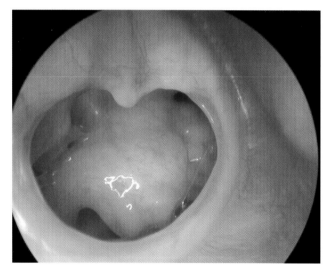

Fig. 1.7.17 Right ear. Subtotal perforation of the tympanic membrane. Fibrous annulus is still intact, which makes the perforation a central one. Spontaneous closure of the perforation is nearly impossible. Promontory; eustachian tube orifice in the superior–anterior part of the promontory. Round window niche posteroinferior to the promontory is visible

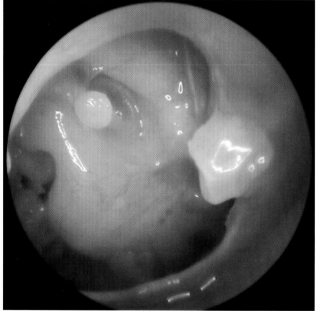

Fig. 1.7.19 Right ear. Nearly total tympanic membrane perforation. Through the perforation promontory, the round window niche can be seen; posterosuperior to the promontory stapes, the head of the stapes, footplate, and above the stapes the facial nerve canal are clearly visible

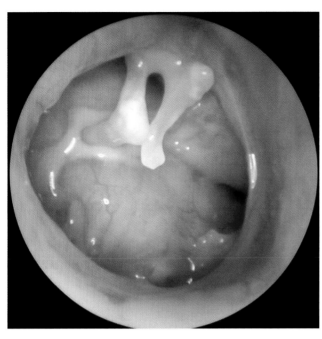

Fig. 1.7.20 Right ear. Nearly total tympanic membrane perforation. Short process of the malleus, malleus handle, long process of the incus, incudostapedial joint, stapes, and posterior crus of the stapes are seen. The mucopurulent material is seen around the footplate and in the round window niche

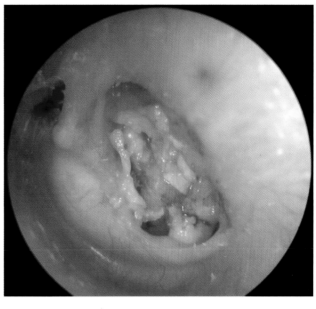

Fig. 1.7.22 Left ear. Marginal perforation of the tympanic membrane in the posterior part. The remnant of the tympanic membrane is opaque and thickened. Ivory-colored cholesteatoma mass is filling the whole middle ear cavity

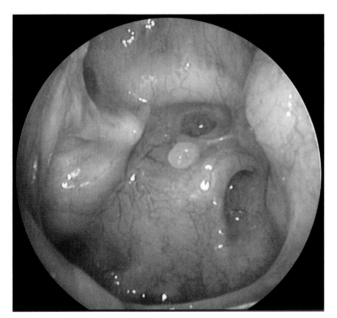

Fig. 1.7.21 Left ear. Nearly total tympanic membrane perforation. Posterior to the promontory, round window niche; posterosuperior to the promontory, stapes, footplate, and stapes tendon; above the stapes, facial nerve canal; and in the anterosuperior part of the middle ear, tensor tympani muscle are seen

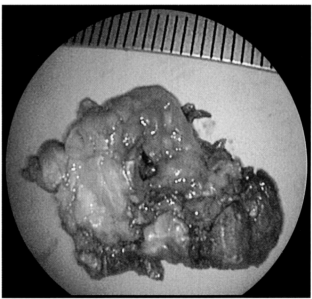

Fig. 1.7.23 A cholesteatoma mass removed from the ear, measuring approximately 4 cm in diameter

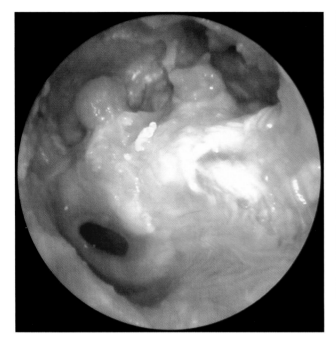

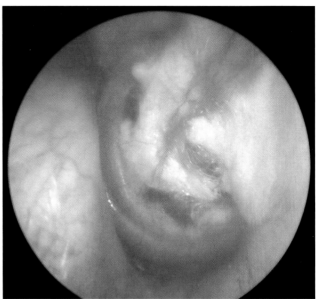

Fig. 1.7.26 Left ear. After myringoplasty the grafted tympanic membrane is very well vascularized. In the anterior part the fibrous annulus and membrane remnant are seen

Fig. 1.7.24 Left ear. Atticoantrotomy cavity after keratin debris has been cleaned. The head of the malleus and the short process of the incus are seen in the cavity. There is a central perforation of 2 mm in the anteroinferior part of the tympanic membrane

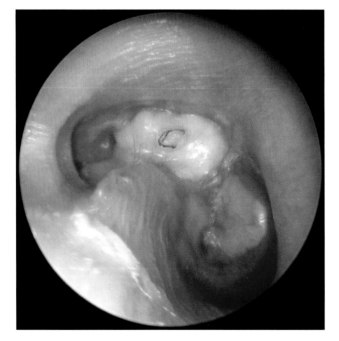

Fig. 1.7.25 Right ear. View after Bondy mastoidectomy. The tympanic membrane is slightly vascularized and retracted. The cholesteatoma is marsupialized into the external ear canal by the atticoantrotomy operation. Bondy mastoidectomy is performed in cases of cholesteatoma that develop from the attic region and extend to the antrum cavity. Since the cholesteatoma mass does not extend into the middle ear cavity, there is no need to open the middle ear cavity. The cholesteatoma is followed and marsupialized into the external ear canal

1.8

Facial Nerve Paralysis

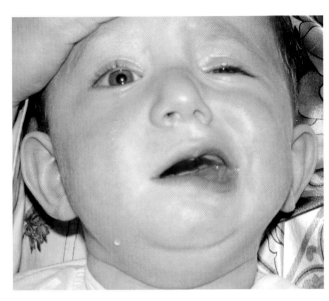

Fig. 1.8.1 Facial nerve paralysis due to facial nerve absence at birth (Courtesy of TESAV)

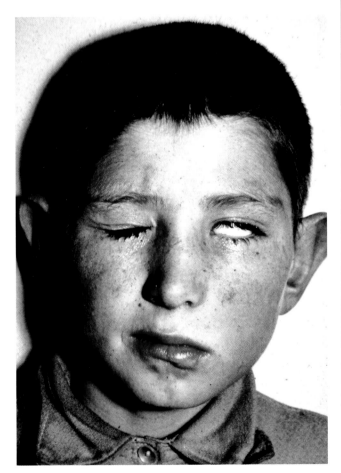

Fig. 1.8.2 Bell's palsy. When the patient closes his eyes, the eye on the paralyzed side rolls up (Courtesy of TESAV)

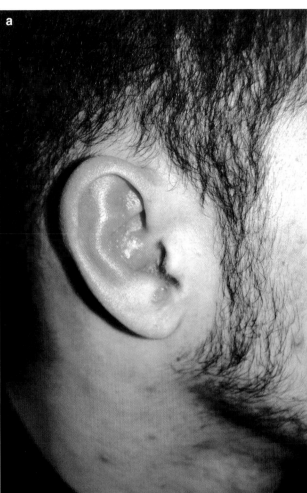

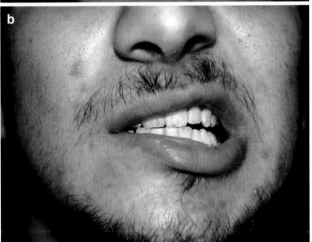

Fig. 1.8.3 Ramsey Hunt syndrome. (a) Vesicles in the right auricle. (b) Right-sided facial nerve paralysis; temporal MR image shows enhancement of the right facial nerve denoting viral infection of the facial nerve (courtesy of Dr. Sarac)

Table 1.8.1 Branches of the facial nerve

Origin	Nerve	Function	Type
Geniculate ganglion	N. petrosus superficialis major	Lacrimation	Parasympathetic
Pyramidal segment	N. stapedius	Contraction of stapes muscle	Motor
Vertical segment	N. chorda tympani	Taste for the anterior two-thirds of the tongue salivation for sublingual and submandibular salivary glands	Sensorial parasympathetic

Table 1.8.2 Staging of nerve injury

Severity	Pathology	Recovery	Sequela
Neuropraxia	Only edema, temporary block in axon flow	Complete	None
Axonotmesis	Myelin sheath degeneration, block in axonal flow	Nearly complete	None
Neurotmesis	Damage to the endo-, peri-, or epineurium	Not always, incomplete	Recovery (if it occurs) with sequela

Table 1.8.3 Causes for intratemporal facial nerve paralysis

Congenital
Traumatic
Infectious
Acute
Chronic
Herpes zoster
Neoplasms
Glomus jugulare
Acoustic neurinoma
Bell paralysis (Bell's palsy)
Other
Sarcoidosis
Polyneuropathy

Table 1.8.4 Topographic tests

Schirmer	Lacrimation
Stapes reflex	Contraction of stapes muscle
Taste	Taste for anterior two-thirds of the tongue
Salivation	The amount of salivation of submandibular gland

1.9

Complications of Otitis Media

The aditus ad antrum connects the attic and middle ear to the mastoid cavity. Since it is a narrow passage, any inflammation may cause mucosal edema and thickening which in turn blocks the aditus ad antrum. Purulent material collects in the mastoid cells. This purulent material applies pressure on the mucosal veins and causes anoxia and acidosis. Acidosis leads to decalcification. Osteoclasts come into the field and remove decalcified bony lamella. All mastoid cells coalesce and make one mastoid cavity. This stage is called the coalescence stage and is the first danger sign of important complications.

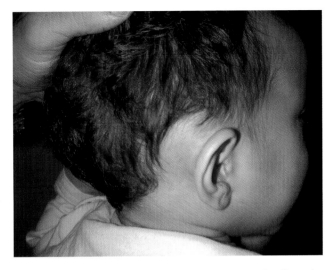

Fig. 1.9.2 Acute mastoiditis during acute otitis media. Note the pinna was pushed anteriorly and laterally. The postauricular sulcus disappeared

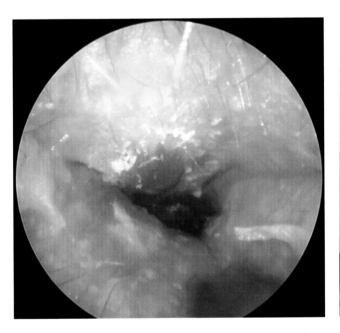

Fig. 1.9.1 Sagging in the posterosuperior wall of the external ear canal in an acute mastoiditis patient

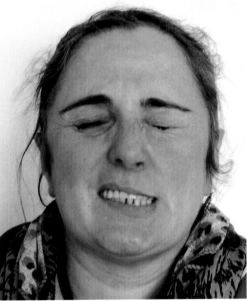

Fig. 1.9.3 Right peripheral facial nerve paresis following acute mastoiditis

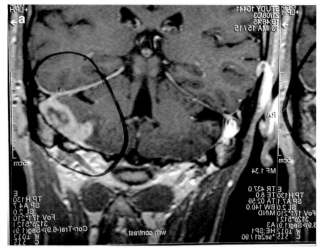

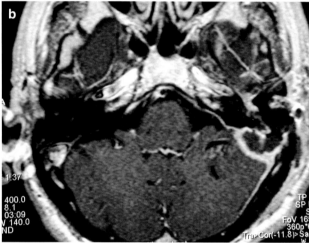

Fig. 1.9.4 Right temporal lobe abscess in a chronic otitis media patient with cholesteatoma. (**a**) Coronal view, (**b**) axial view

Table 1.9.1 Complications of middle ear infections

Extracranial
Acute mastoiditis
Facial nerve paralysis
Acute suppurative labyrinthitis
Petrositis
Intracranial
Meningitis
Intracranial abscess
Extradural abscess
Subdural abscess
Brain abscess
Lateral sinus thrombophlebitis
Otitic hydrocephalus

Table 1.9.2 Main symptoms in otogenic complications

Disease	Fever	Neurologic findings	CSF findings
Mastoiditis	+++	−	−
Petrositis	++	+	−
Lateral sinus thrombophlebitis[a]	+++	−	−
Otitic hydrocephalus	−	±	Pressure over 300
Bacterial meningitis	+++	+	+
Extradural abscess	±	−	−
Subdural abscess	+	±	−
Brain abscess	+	+	+

[a] Chills are a highly diagnostic symptom associated with lateral sinus thrombophlebitis

1.10

Hearing Loss

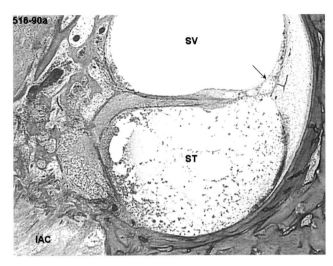

Fig. 1.10.1 Inflammation in the labyrinth of a patient with total hearing loss following suppurative labyrinthitis (courtesy of Paparella, Paparella otopathology lab director)

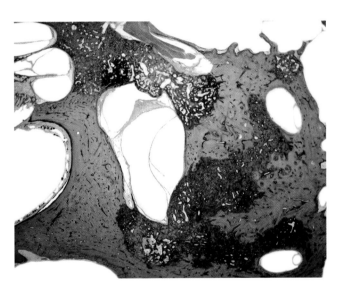

Fig. 1.10.2 Temporal bone section. Otosclerosis causing obstruction in the vestibular aqueduct and endolymphatic hydrops in all turns of the cochlea (courtesy of Paparella, Paparella otopathology lab director)

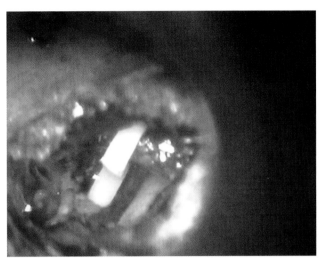

Fig. 1.10.3 In stapes surgery, the stapes suprastructure is removed and a hole is created in the footplate for a Teflon piston. The Teflon piston is placed in the footplate and hung on the long process of the incus which creates a bridge instead of the stapes (courtesy of Sennaroğlu)

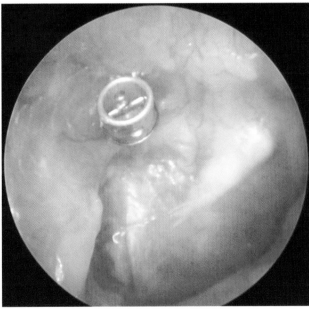

Fig. 1.10.4 Extruded metal piston in the external auditory canal in a patient who had undergone otosclerosis surgery in the past

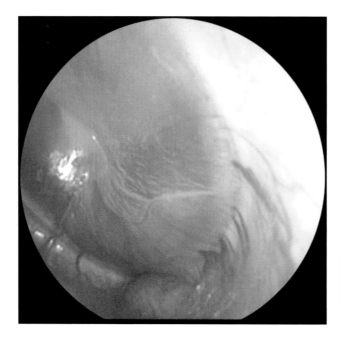

Fig. 1.10.5 Glomus jugulare. A *pink–bluish* silhouette of a glomus tumor behind the tympanic membrane

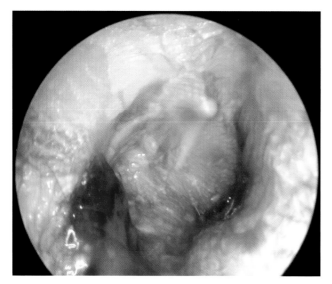

Fig. 1.10.6 Glomus jugulare tumor extending out to the external auditory canal

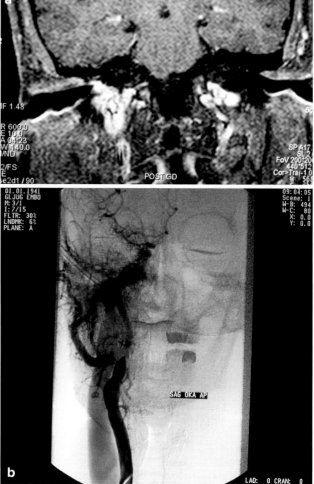

Fig. 1.10.7 (**a**) Temporal MR image. Glomus jugulare tumor on the right side extending to the hypotympanum. (**b**) Angiography shows hypervascularized glomus tumor

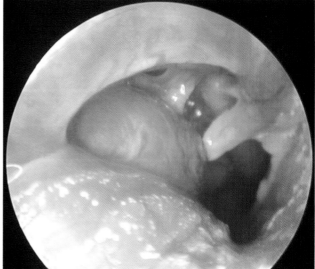

Fig. 1.10.8 Right ear. Through the tympanic membrane perforation, the glomus tumor is seen to be localized in the hypotympanum. It is in contact with the incudostapedial joint

Table 1.10.1 Etiology of hearing losses

Cause	Conductive hearing loss	Sensorineural hearing loss
Congenital	Ear atresia	Prenatal
	Ossicular pathologies	Genetic
		Pregnancy
		Rubella
Acquired	External ear canal	Birth (hypoxia jaundice)
	Wax	Trauma (iatrogenic, acoustic trauma, head trauma)
	Foreign body	
	Middle ear	Inflammatory (chronic otitis media, mumps, meningitis)
	Otitis media with effusion	
	Chronic otitis media	Degenerative presbyacusis
	Otosclerosis	Ototoxicity
	Traumatic drum	Neoplastic acoustic neurinoma
	Perforations	Idiopathic Meniere disease
		Sudden hearing loss

Table 1.10.2 Ototoxic drugs

Salicylic acid
Aminoglycosides
Streptomycin
Dihydrostreptomycin
Neomycin
Gentamycin
Kanamysin
Tobramycin
Diuretics
Furosemide
Etacrynic acid
Chemotherapeutic agents
Cisplatin/carboplatin
Nitrogen mustard
6-Amino nicotinamide
Vincristine/vinblastine
Misonidazole
Dichloro-methotroxate
Lonidamine
Paclitaxel
Others
Vancomycin
Polymyxin B
Iodoform
Tetanus antitoxin
Interferon alpha 2a

EAR
NOSE
THROAT AND NECK

1.11

Otalgia

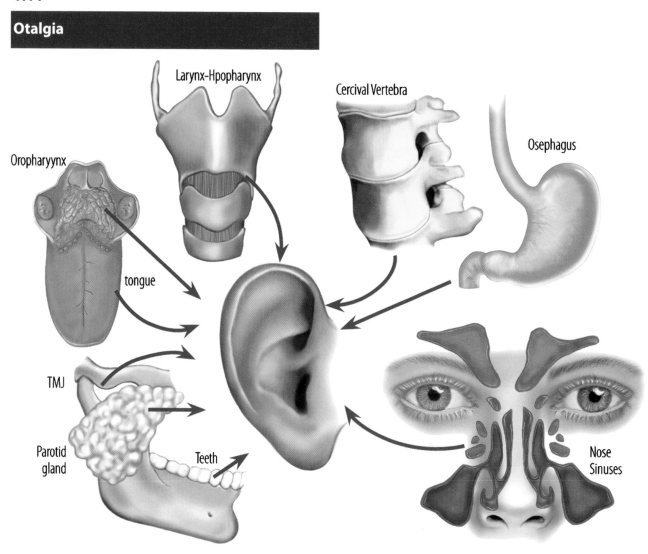

Fig. 1.11.1 Nonotological causes of earache. The most common cause of otalgia is dental problems in adults

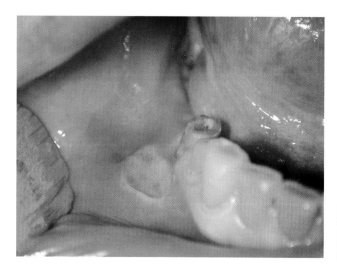

Fig. 1.11.2 Aphthous stomatitis behind the molar teeth in the gingivobuccal sulcus may cause severe ear pain

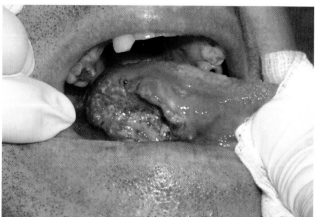

Fig. 1.11.3 Squamous cell carcinoma of the tongue which has caused ear pain

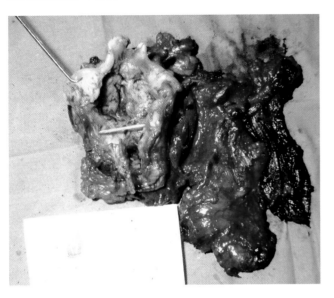

Fig. 1.11.4 Earache may also be seen in laryngeal carcinomas

1.12

Temporal Bone Fractures

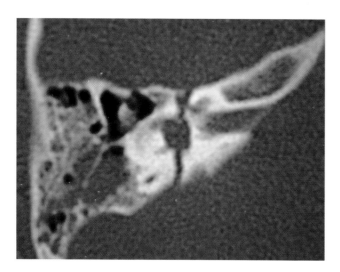

Fig. 1.12.1 Axial CT scan. Transverse temporal bone fracture on the left side. High-resolution CT scans of the temporal bone provide necessary information about the fracture. Audiometric examination helps in the diagnosis

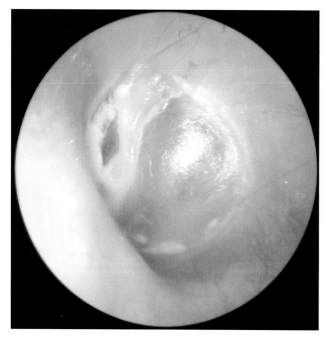

Fig. 1.12.2 In longitudinal fractures, a fracture line at the posterosuperior part of the external ear canal may be seen

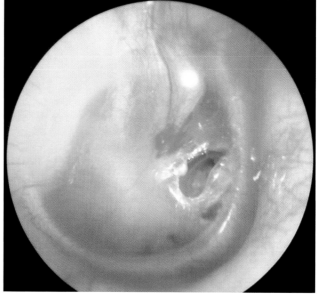

Fig. 1.12.3 Traumatic tympanic membrane perforation. These perforations are sometimes seen after a blow to the ear. To be sure that the perforation is really traumatic, the physician should check that the edges of the perforation are irregular and hemorrhagic

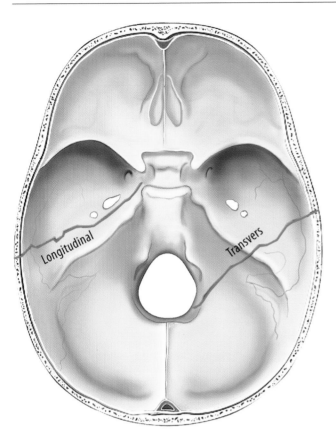

Fig. 1.12.4 Schematic representation of longitudinal and transverse fractures. Temporal bone fractures are classified into two main groups: longitudinal and transverse fractures. Longitudinal fractures are much more frequent, with the incidence of longitudinal fractures being four times greater than transverse fractures. Generally, temporal and parietal blows are associated with longitudinal fractures. Since the areas of the foramina are relatively weaker parts of the skull base, fractures tend to occur in their vicinity. Longitudinal fractures start in the squamous portion and go to the middle ear through the posterior and superior walls of the external ear canal and then to the petrous apex. Generally, conductive hearing loss is accompanied by longitudinal temporal bone fractures. Facial nerve injury may occur at the geniculate ganglion area and is only seen in 15% of longitudinal fractures. Tympanic membrane perforation or bleeding into the middle ear may also be seen. Transverse fractures generally occur due to frontal or occipital trauma. Since the blow comes from anterior-posterior or posterior-anterior direction, the fracture line occurs at a right angle to the axis of the petrous bone and the fracture line starts from the foramen magnum or jugular foramen and extends to the middle ear. It frequently affects the facial nerve and inner ear. Hemotympanum may be associated with transverse fractures, but tympanic membrane perforation is not seen. Temporal bone fractures do not always follow these general guidelines, and some fractures are mixed. These fractures are evaluated according to the type of lesion

How to Make the Diagnosis of CSF Draining from the External Ear Canal

If the fluid is collected on a filtered paper or on a gauze, it forms a halo around the circle of blood. If the fluid can be collected in a tube, beta-2 transferrin positivity indicates CSF leak.

Table 1.12.1 How to treat CSF fistula

Head is elevated 30°
Gaita softeners are prescribed
Diuretics such as diazomide are given to decrease the CSF pressure
Wide-spectrum antibiotics are started as prophylaxis against meningitis
No packing is done to the external ear canal

Table 1.12.2 Differential diagnosis between longitudinal and transverse temporal fractures

	Longitudinal	Transverse
Frequency (approximate %)	80	20
Hearing loss	Conductive	Sensorineural
Vertigo	Rare	Frequent
Facial nerve paralysis	Rare (10–15%)	Frequent (50%)

1.13

Tinnitus

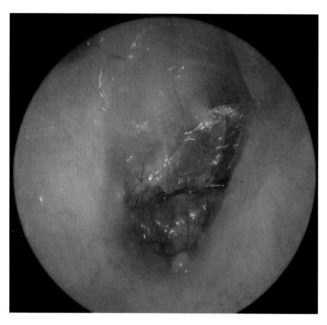

Fig. 1.13.1 Wax filling the ear canal may cause tinnitus

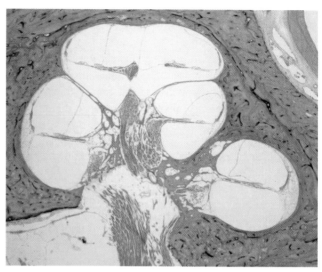

Fig. 1.13.3 Hydropic Reissner's membrane in all turns of the cochlea (courtesy of Paparella, Paparella otopathology lab director). Endolymphatic hydrops causes roaring-type tinnitus

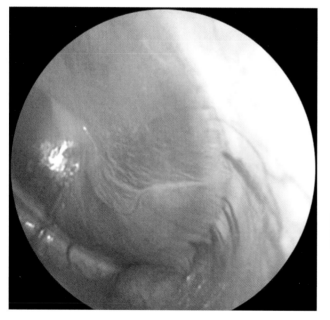

Fig. 1.13.2 Glomus jugulare tumor causing objective tinnitus

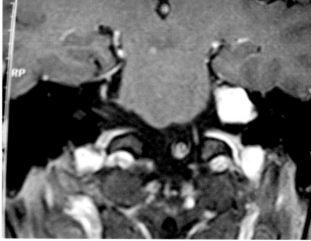

Fig. 1.13.4 Acoustic neuroma on the left side. Unilateral tinnitus, if associated with high-frequency hearing loss and low scores of speech discrimination, should be investigated for acoustic neurinoma

Tinnitus is any abnormal noise in the ear. It may be objective or subjective. All pathologies in the external, middle, and inner ear may cause tinnitus. Unilateral tinnitus, if associated with high-frequency hearing loss, should be investigated and acoustic neurinoma eliminated.

Objective tinnitus can be heard by the examiner as well. Objective tinnitus is rare and the commonest form is vascular pathology such as glomus jugulare tumor, high jugular bulbus, arteriovenous malformations, and carotid body tumors. The normal pulsatile noise of blood passing through the internal carotid artery may also cause tinnitus. If you close the ear it becomes more apparent. Temporomandibular joint pathologies, insects in the external ear canal, and palatal myoclonus are other pathological conditions causing objective tinnitus besides vascular causes. Most forms of objective tinnitus are readily identifiable and curable.

Table 1.13.2 Ear diseases associated with objective tinnitus

Vascular pathologies
Arteriovenous malformation
Aneurysms
Carotid body tumor
Glomus jugulare
Palatal myoclonus
TMJ pathologies
Insects in the external ear canal

Table 1.13.1 Ear diseases associated with subjective tinnitus

External ear	Wax
	Foreign body
Middle ear	Chronic otitis media
	Otosclerosis
	Otitis media with effusion
	Ossicular chain pathologies
Inner ear	Presbyacusis
	Acoustic trauma
	Ototoxic drugs
	Meniere's disease
	Acoustic neuroma

Table 1.13.3 Drugs that can cause or exacerbate tinnitus

Aspirin
Aminoglycosides
Loop diuretics
Quinine
Indomethacin
Alcohol

1.14

Vertigo

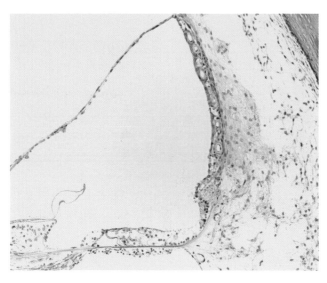

Fig. 1.14.1 Normal appearance of Reissner's membrane and the tectorial membrane (courtesy of Paparella, Paparella otopathology lab director)

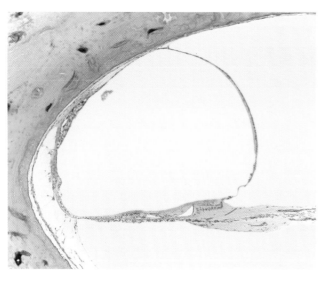

Fig. 1.14.2 Hydropic Reissner's membrane in one turn of the cochlea (courtesy of Paparella, Paparella otopathology lab director)

Table 1.14.1 Anamnesis in vertigo patient

Onset of vertigo
Character of vertigo, real vertigo, or dizziness
Duration
Relationship to the movements of the head
Other associated symptoms, tinnitus, hearing loss etc.

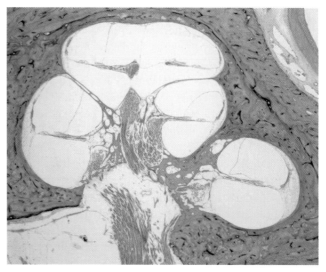

Fig. 1.14.3 Profound endolymphatic hydrops in all turns of the cochlea (courtesy of Paparella, Paparella otopathology lab director)

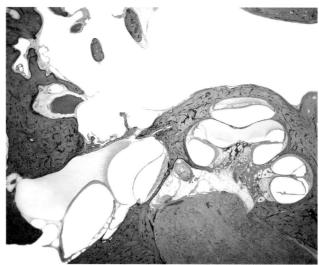

Fig. 1.14.4 Intracanalicular acoustic neuroma and serous labyrinthitis in the vestibule and cochlea (courtesy of Paparella, Paparella otopathology lab director)

Table 1.14.2 Differential diagnosis in vertigo according to duration

Duration	No hearing loss	With hearing loss
Seconds	Benign paroxysmal positional vertigo	
Minutes	Vertebrobasilar insufficiency	
Hours		Endolymphatic hydrops (Meniere disease)
Days	Vestibular neuritis	Labyrinthitis
Weeks	Intracranial pathologies Multiple sclerosis	Acoustic neurinoma, psychogenic

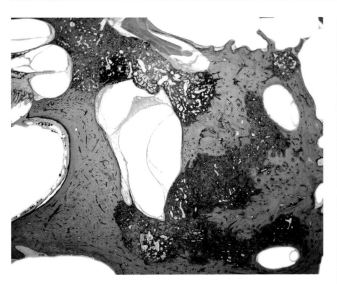

Fig. 1.14.5 Temporal bone section. Otosclerosis causing obstruction in the vestibular aqueduct and endolymphatic hydrops in all turns of the cochlea (courtesy of Paparella, Paparella otopathology lab director)

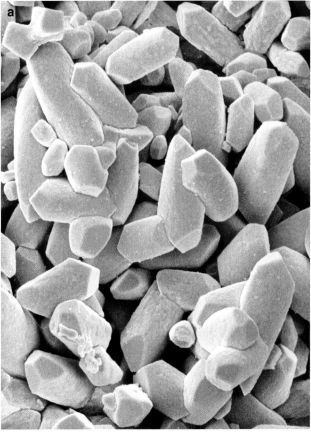

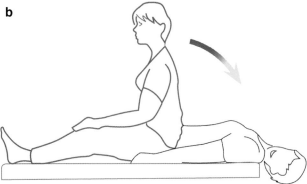

Fig. 1.14.6 (a) Balancing stone from inner ear. Color scanning electron micrograph of crystals of calcium carbonate on the surface of an otolith. An otolith or *otoconium* is a calcified stone that is found in the otolith organs of the inner ear. They are attached to sensory hairs, and, when the head tilts, the movement of the stones causes nerve impulses that form the basis of the sense of balance. In humans, otoconia can range in size from 3 to 30 μm (millionths of a meter) across (visual photos). (b) Dix Hallpike maneuver. The patient is brought to the supine position from the sitting position with the head turned to one side. The maneuver is repeated on the opposite side. The presence of nystagmus or any feeling of movement is recorded

Table 1.14.3 Differential diagnosis in central and peripheral vertigo

	Peripheral	Central
Unsteadiness	Slight, moderate	Severe
Nausea, vomiting	Severe	Slight
Hearing symptoms	Frequent	Rare
Neurologic symptoms	Rare	Frequent
Compensation	Fast	Slow

Table 1.14.4 Differential diagnosis in central and peripheral positional vertigo

	Peripheral	Central
Latent period	+	−
Adaptation	+	−
Fatigue	+	−

Fig. 1.14.7 Epley maneuver for benign paroxysmal positional vertigo (BPPV). The patient is brought to the Dix Hallpike position, with the head turned 45° to the affected side. The head is then turned to the opposite side. The patient's head is held in each position for 30 seconds. The whole body and head is brought to the lateral decubitus position. The patient is brought to the starting position-sitting position

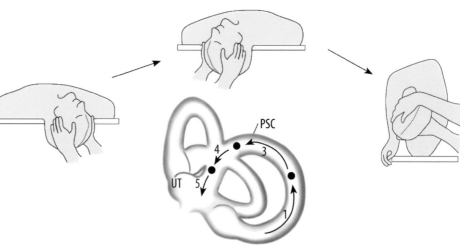

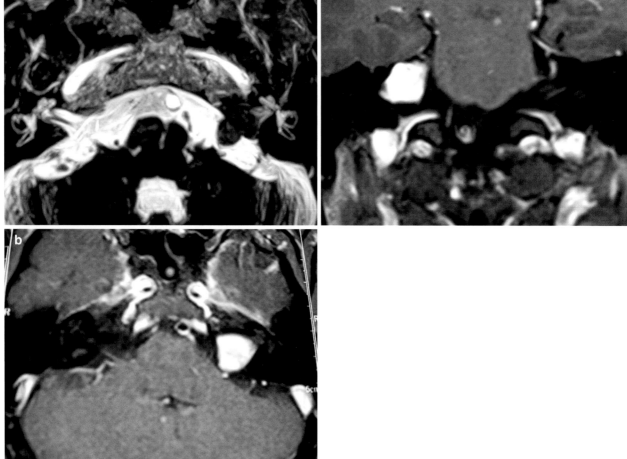

Fig. 1.14.8 (**a-c**) Acoustic neuroma on the right side. MR imaging is particularly useful in diagnosing acoustic neuroma. The lesions enhance with gadolinium injection

NOSE

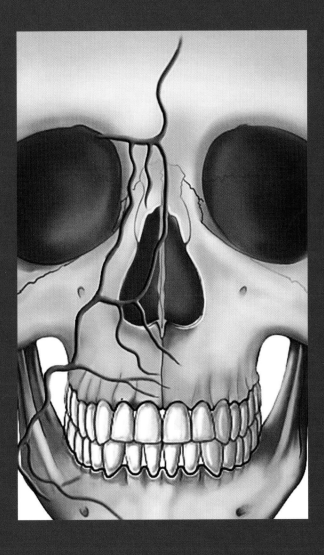

CONTENTS

T. Metin Önerci: *Diagnosis in Otorhinolaryngology*
DOI: 10.1007/978-3-642-00499-5_2, © Springer-Verlag Berlin Heidelberg 2009

2.1

The Common Cold and the Flu

Both the flu and the common cold are respiratory illnesses caused by different viruses. The flu is an infection of the respiratory system caused by the influenza virus, the common cold is caused mainly by rhinoviruses. Common cold/acute viral rhinosinusitis is defined as duration of symptoms for less than 10 days. Acute nonviral rhinosinusitis is defined as an increase of symptoms after 5 days or persistent symptoms after 10 days with less than 12 weeks' duration.

Although the symptoms are similar and it is difficult to tell the difference between the common cold and the flu based on symptoms alone, the flu is worse than the common cold. There is usually fever (temperature above 39°C), and symptoms such as headache, body aches, extreme tiredness, sore throat, and dry cough are more common and intense. The symptoms appear suddenly. People with colds are more likely to have a runny or stuffy nose. Colds generally do not result in serious health problems, such as pneumonia, bacterial infections, or hospitalizations. Adults get an average of two to four colds per year, mostly between September and May. Young children suffer from an average of six to eight colds per year. People recover from the common cold in 1 week; however, recovery from the flu may take more than 1 week, especially for the elderly, who may feel weak for a long time even after symptoms resolve.

Nonsteroidal anti-inflammatory drugs (NSAIDs) can be used. However, acetaminophen, aspirin, or any other NSAIDs may worsen asthma and/or peptic ulcers. Aspirin should not be used in children younger than 18 years because it may play a role in causing Reye syndrome, a rare but severe liver and central nervous system condition. Congestion, cough, and nasal discharge may be treated with a decongestant, antihistamine, or a combination of the two. Some people such as those with thyroid disease or high blood pressure should not take decongestants. There are no antiviral medications available for treating the common cold. Antibiotics are not useful for treating a cold, and should only be taken to treat bacterial complications that arise from it.

Other Remedies

Herbs and minerals such as echinacea, eucalyptus, garlic, honey, lemon, menthol, zinc, and vitamin C have received extensive publicity as cold remedies. However, none of these claims is solidly supported by scientific studies.

Adequate liquid intake (eight glasses of water and/or juice per day) is recommended to prevent dehydration. Coffee, tea, or cola drinks that contain caffeine and any drinks that contain alcohol should be avoided to prevent their dehydration effects. Smoking should be stopped. Since inhaling smoke of other smokers will cause more irritation in the throat and will increase coughing, patients should stay away from other smokers.

Bed rest is helpful for recovery. Until the symptoms are gone, it is not advisable to go back to full activity. In the treatment of the flu, antiviral medications may be used. They may reduce the duration of the disease if started early. Oseltamivir or zanamivir may be used to treat the influenza virus. Oseltamivir or zanamivir given within 2 days of the appearance of flu symptoms will reduce the length of the illness and the severity of symptoms by at least 1 day. Early treatment can lead to faster recovery.

Flu Vaccines May Help to Prevent Getting the Flu

There are currently two vaccine options: the flu shot and the nasal spray vaccine. The shot gives more reliable protection and the spray is recommended only for non-high-risk groups.

The best tool for preventing the flu is the flu vaccine, and the best time to get a flu vaccine is from early October to mid-November. The vaccine can also be given at any point during the flu season, even if the virus has already begun to spread in the community. A flu vaccine should be repeated every year because the virus is constantly changing and new vaccines are developed annually to protect against new strains.

Table 2.1.1 Who should get a flu vaccine?

Adults 50 years or older
All children under 5 years of age (only after 6 months of age)
Adults and children aged 2–64 years with chronic medical conditions, especially asthma, other lung diseases, and heart disease
All women who will be pregnant during the influenza season
Residents of nursing homes and other chronic care facilities
Health-care workers involved in direct patient care

Table 2.1.2 Contraindications to flu vaccination

Egg allergy
History of Guillain-Barre syndrome
Acute illness or fever

Table 2.1.3 Clinical features of the common cold and flu

	Common cold	**Flu**
Virus	Rhinovirus	Influenza
Contagiousness	Droplets by inhalation or touch	Droplets by inhalation
Onset	1–3 days after virus entrance	Sudden
Duration	One week	One week or more
Frequency	Children six to eight colds per year, adults two to four colds per year	Once
Symptoms	Milder	Worse
	Weakened senses of taste and smell, cough, runny or stuffy nose, sneezing, scratchy throat	Fever (39°C or above), body aches, extreme tiredness, dry cough more common, headache, sore throat, chills, tiredness
Complications	No serious complications	May have serious complications, pneumonia, bacterial infections
		May be fatal in elderly, immunocompromised, and chronically ill patients
Treatment	Acetaminophen	Acetaminophen
	Antihistamine and/or decongestant	Antihistamine and/or decongestant
	Adequate fluid intake (eight glasses of water or juice)	Adequate fluid intake (eight glasses of water or juice)
	Avoid smoking and alcohol	Avoid smoking and alcohol
	Avoid caffeine and alcohol	Avoid caffeine and alcohol
	No antibiotics	No antibiotics

Table 2.1.4 How to prevent a cold

Close contact with people who have a cold should be avoided especially during the first few days when they are most likely to spread the infection
Hands should be washed after touching someone who has a cold
Fingers should be kept away from the nose and the eyes to avoid self-infecting the cold virus particles
A second hand towel should be put in the bathroom for healthy people to use
The environment should be humidified
The nose and the mouth should be covered with a tissue when coughing or sneezing

EAR

NOSE

THROAT AND NECK

2.2

Rhinitis

Rhinitis is a clinical diagnosis and is defined as inflammation of the nasal mucosa with one or more symptoms of sneezing, itching, rhinorrhea, and nasal blockage lasting for at least 1 h on most days. All diseases causing rhinorrhea and nasal obstruction should be considered in the differential diagnosis of rhinitis.

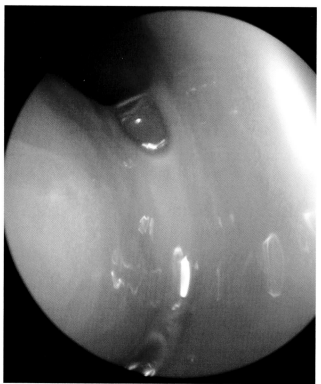

Fig. 2.2.3 Upper respiratory tract infection, 6th day, mucoid nasal discharge

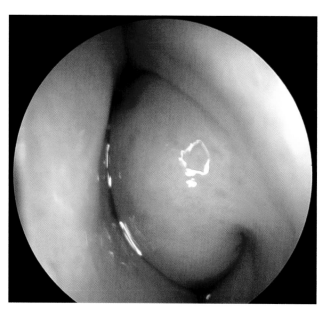

Fig. 2.2.1 Allergic rhinitis. Serous nasal discharge with hypertrophic, pale inferior turbinates

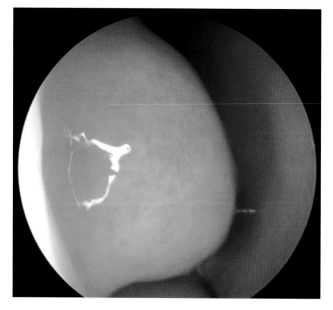

Fig. 2.2.2 Acute rhinitis, early period. Right inferior turbinate mucosa is hyperemic and there is serous secretion

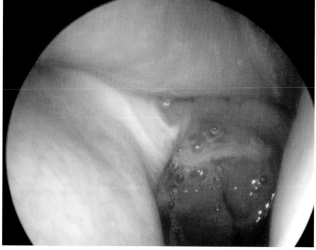

Fig. 2.2.4 Right acute maxillary sinusitis. Purulent nasal discharge with draining to the nasopharynx through the middle meatus

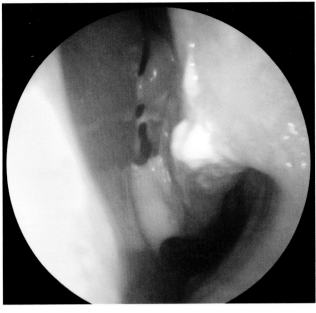

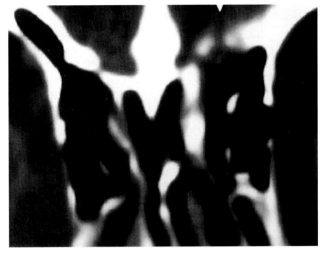

Fig. 2.2.7 Cerebrospinal fluid (CSF) rhinorrhea. Coronal CT showing fracture line in the fovea ethmoidalis of anterior ethmoid area

Fig. 2.2.5 Chronic sinusitis, purulent discharge in left nasal cavity

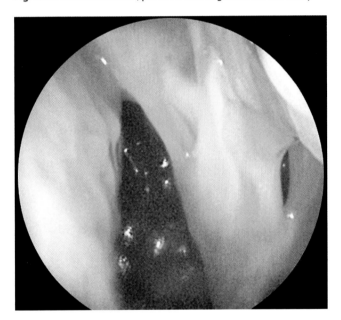

Fig. 2.2.6 Eosinophilic mucin in a patient with nonallergic rhinitis with eosinophilia syndrome (NARES). The discharge is sticky, thick, and *yellow-green*

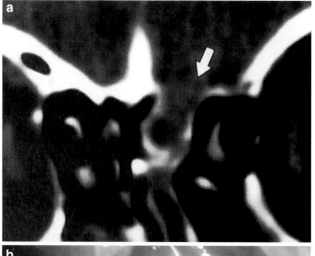

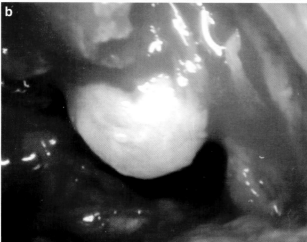

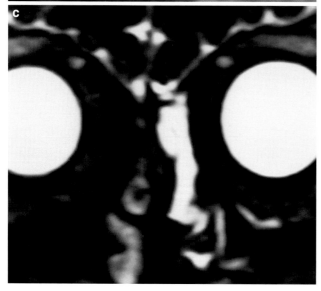

Fig. 2.2.8 CSF rhinorrhea. **(a)** Coronal CT showing herniation through lamina cribrosa at the anterior ethmoid area (*arrow*). **(b)** Photograph of the herniated tissue. **(c)** MR cisternography; CSF leak is seen

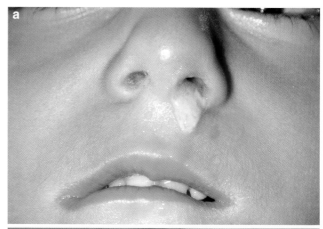

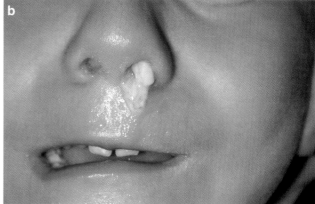

Fig. 2.2.9 Nasal foreign body. **(a)** Unilateral left-sided purulent nasal discharge; the patient presented with a 1-month history of foul odor. **(b)** Foreign body, a piece of tissue, is seen in the left nostril during removal. Generally young children insert foreign bodies into their noses. A unilateral nasal discharge in children should raise the suspicion of a foreign body. Foul smell can be noticed in patients if the foreign body is present for a long period of time. To remove the foreign body, the child should be immobilized. The limbs may be wrapped in a linen cloth and the head kept immobile. Ithar sonde may be used to remove the foreign body. Its blunt curved end passes behind the foreign body and is then taken out. General anesthesia may be given in certain situations, since attempts at removal may push the object to the nasopharynx with the risk of inhalation

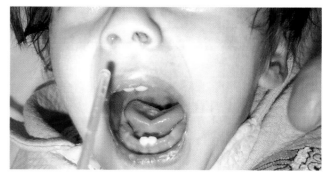

Fig. 2.2.10 A rubber foreign material in the left nasal passage. The child should be kept immobile during removal of the foreign body. To remove the foreign material, a curved instrument with a blunt tip should be used such as Ithar sonde or ear curette

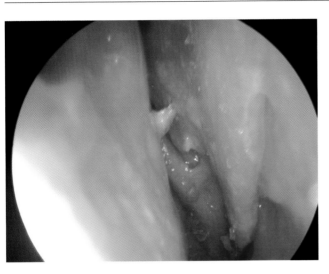

Fig. 2.2.11 Atrophic rhinitis. Atrophy of the nasal mucosa and turbinates with *yellow-green* copious foul-smelling crusts filling the nasal cavity

Table 2.2.1 Classification of rhinitis[a]

Allergic
Seasonal
Perennial
Infectious
Acute
Chronic
Specific
Nonspecific
Nonallergic
Eosinophilic rhinitis (NARES – nonallergic rhinitis with eosinophilia syndrome)
Others
Occupational
Hormonal
Drug induced
Irritants
Emotional
Food (gustatory rhinitis)
Atrophic
Geriatric
Idiopathic

[a]International Consensus Report on the Diagnosis and Management of Rhinitis 1994

Nonallergic rhinitis with eosinophilia syndrome (NARES) is a type of rhinitis associated with the symptoms of perennial rhinitis without any identifiable allergen hypersensitivity. IgE-mediated mechanisms do not play a role. Excessive eosinophilia is demonstrated in nasal secretions. Nonallergic asthma and analgesic intolerance are more common in these patients. The etiology is unclear. They often respond well to treatment with intranasal corticosteroids.

Occupational rhinitis arises in response to an airborne agent present in the workplace. Causes include laboratory animals, hair (hairdressers), grain (bakers and agricultural workers), wood dusts, latex, and chemicals.

Hormonal rhinitis can occur during pregnancy, puberty, and also in hypothyroidism and acromegaly. Postmenopausal hormonal changes may also cause atrophic nasal pathologies.

Emotional rhinitis is the result of emotional factors such as stress and sexual arousal due to autonomic stimulation as in honeymoon rhinitis.

Gustatory rhinorrhea occurs when eating hot and spicy foods. True food allergy never produces isolated rhinitis symptoms. Hypersensitivity reactions to colorants and preservatives in the food may also occur.

The term idiopathic rhinitis is generally used instead of vasomotor rhinitis. Vasomotor rhinitis is a subgroup of NARES, which is thought to be due to an imbalance of autonomic nervous supply and peptidergic nervous mechanisms. Engorged blood vessels lead to nasal obstruction. These patients present with nasal hyperresponsiveness to nonspecific stimuli such as strong smells, irritants such as exhaust fumes, or environmental temperature. Nonimmunologic stimuli such as cold air can degranulate mast cells with mediator release and may cause the symptoms.

Atrophic rhinitis is characterized by progressive atrophy of the underlying bone of the turbinates and nasal mucosa. Copious foul-smelling crusts fill the nasal cavity. The patient complains of hyposmia, nasal congestion, and constant bad smell in the nose. *Klebsiella ozaenae* is generally found in the nasal cavity of these patients.

Table 2.2.2 Differential diagnosis of rhinitis

Polyps
Mechanical factors
Septum deviation
Turbinate hypertrophy
Adenoidal hypertrophy
Foreign bodies
Choanal atresia
Tumors
Benign
Malignant
Granulomas
Wegener granulomatosis
Sarcoidosis
Infectious
Tuberculosis
Lepra
Malignant midline destructive granuloma
CSF fistula

Table 2.2.3 Diagnostic tests for rhinitis

Skin prick tests
Specific IgE measurements
Nasal smear
Nasal provocation tests
Histamine/methacholine
Allergen
Rhinomanometry
Acoustic rhinometry
CT, MR imaging
Biopsy, electron microscopic examination
Sweat test

Table 2.2.4 Drugs that can induce rhinitis

Antihypertensives
Reserpine
Guanethidine
Phentolamine
Methyldopa
ACE inhibitors
Alpha adrenoreceptor antagonists
Topical ophthalmic beta blockers
Chlorpromazine
Aspirin
Nonsteroidal anti-inflammatory agents
Oral contraceptives
Topical decongestants (rhinitis medicamentosa – long-term use of cocaine and nasal drops or sprays)

Table 2.2.5 Diagnostic features of noninfectious rhinitis

	Seasonal	Perennial	Perennial nonallergic
Time of year	Seasonal	Perennial	Perennial
Age of onset	10–20	10–20	Adulthood
Prominent symptom	Rhinorrhea, sneezing, itching	Rhinorrhea, sneezing, itching	Rhinorrhea, blockage
Eye symptoms	Common	Uncommon	Not present
Nasal cytology	EO (Eosinophil)	EO	EO/NT (Neutrophil)
Allergens	Pollens	Dust mite, moulds, animal	Negative
Polyps	Uncommon	Uncommon	Frequent

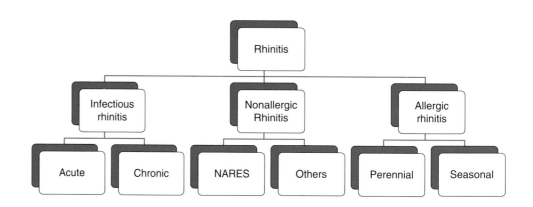

Fig. 2.2.12 Classification of rhinitis

2.3

Allergic Rhinitis

Allergy is an inappropriate and harmful immune response to a normally harmless substance. Generally, allergens are proteins that do not cause any reactions in nonatopic individuals.

What is atopy?

Atopy is an inherited predisposition to produce IgE antibodies to certain substances.

What is the difference between atopy and allergy?

Atopy is the genetic predisposition to produce IgE antibodies. To develop allergy, stimulation of the cells of the immune system to produce IgE antibodies is needed. Although almost 25–30% of the population is atopic, not every atopic person develops allergy. Environmental factors are important in the development of allergic disease.

Allergic Reaction

Allergens enter the body through the airways, the gastrointestinal tract, or the skin. In atopic patients an allergen is recognized as being foreign to the immune system. B cells are stimulated to produce specific IgE antibodies. These IgE antibodies bind to the surface of mast cells. On subsequent exposures, the allergens bind to the IgE antibodies. Bridging two IgE antibodies makes the mast cell degranulate and the mast cell releases histamine and other cytokines that cause allergic reactions.

Early Response

The early response is initiated after bridging of IgE antibodies on the mast cells. Mast cells release mediators such as histamine, prostaglandins, leukotrienes, platelet-activating factor, and bradykinin. These mediators cause vascular dilatation, increased permeability, and attract inflammatory cells into the tissues starting the inflammation. The early response is characterized by sneezing, rhinorrhea, bronchoconstriction, and increased bronchial responsiveness.

Late Response

The mediators released from mast cells attract inflammatory cells such as eosinophils, lymphocytes, neutrophils, and monocytes into the tissues. Therefore, the late response is a cell-mediated response. The late response is characterized by prolonged mucus secretion, edema formation, and bronchial hyperresponsiveness.

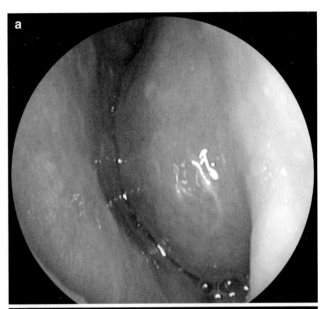

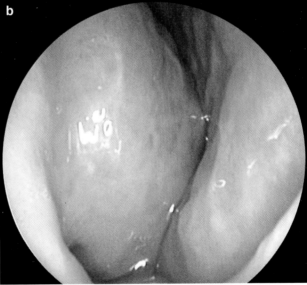

Fig. 2.3.1 (a, b) Allergic rhinitis. The turbinates are *pale, bluish*, and swollen. Watery serous secretion is seen in both nasal passages

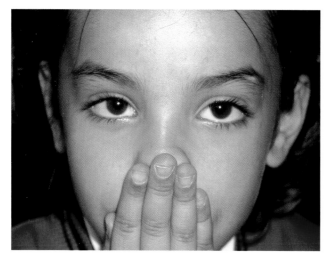

Fig. 2.3.2 Allergy salute is a very common sign of allergic rhinitis in children

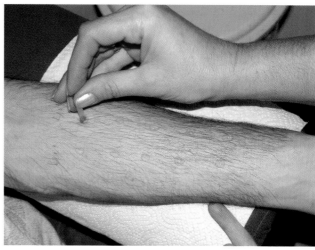

Fig. 2.3.5 Skin prick test

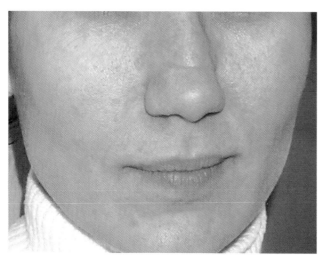

Fig. 2.3.3 Supratip crease. Horizontal line in the supratip area due to repeated use of allergic salute

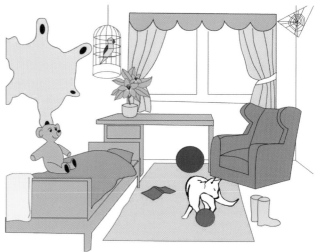

Fig. 2.3.6 Items that should not be present in the room of an allergic child

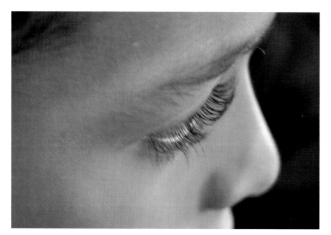

Fig. 2.3.4 Long, silky eyelashes in an allergic child

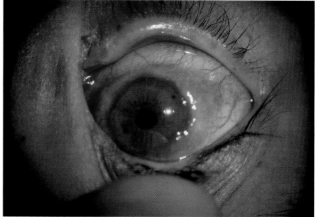

Fig. 2.3.7 Allergic conjunctivitis, erythema, and edema of the conjunctival mucosa, and watering. Limbal elevation can be identified (courtesy of Kıratlı D)

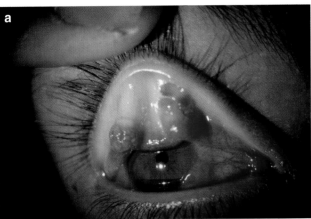

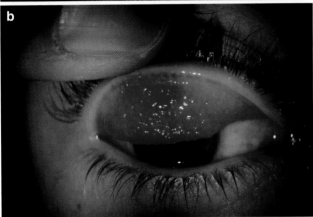

Fig. 2.3.8 (a, b) Giant papillary conjunctivitis, generally seen in patients using contact lenses. Tarsal conjunctiva is sensitized to the allergen adhered to the outer surface of the lens. Due to continuous irritation, the upper tarsal conjunctiva develops giant papillae. The cornea is never involved. Discontinuing lens use together with some topical antiallergic eye drops such as sodium cromoglycate helps the situation (courtesy of Kıratli)

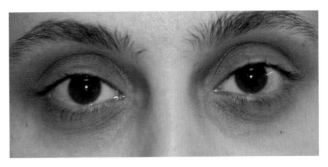

Fig. 2.3.9 Allergic shiners, dark discoloration of the lower lids

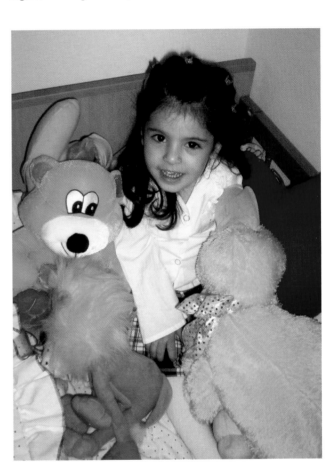

Fig. 2.3.10 Stuffed animals with artificial fur are major dust reservoirs and should not be kept in the room of an allergic child

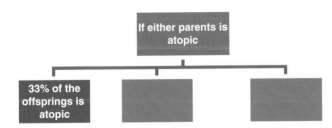

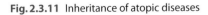

Fig. 2.3.11 Inheritance of atopic diseases

Table 2.3.1 Pollen avoidance

Avoid going on picnics during the pollen season
Wear sunglasses outdoors
Stay inside in the late afternoon[a]
Keep the windows closed in the late afternoon[a]
Keep the windows closed in the car
Use pollen filters if possible

[a]Pollens rise with the heat during the day and come down as the air starts cooling during late afternoon. Therefore, in the late afternoon exposure is highest

Table 2.3.2 Dust mite allergen avoidance[a]

Indoors
Avoid humidity
Avoid warm environment
Ventilate adequately
Reducing the burden of allergens
Avoid wall-to-wall carpeting; tile floors with small rugs are preferable
Remove dust reservoirs such as stuffed animals with artificial fur, soft toys, woollen blankets, old mattresses, silk flowers, mounted animals, books on open shelves, feather pillows or bedding, upholstered furniture
Use pillow covers and mattress covers impermeable to dust mites
Removing the allergens
Superfiltering or HEPA filter vacuum cleaners preferable (at least twice a week)
Clean with a damp cloth every week
Wash the laundry with water hotter than 60°C every week; if possible expose to sunlight

[a]A general understanding of allergy and treatment is important. Fulfilling these measures only partially may not be enough to prevent the symptoms. For example, killing the mites with chemicals may not eradicate the allergen. It may persist for months or even years. Since the mites live in deep pores and attach to the fabric, deep vacuum cleaning is needed to remove the allergen

2.4

Nasal Vestibulitis and Nasal Furunculosis and Mucormycosis

Infection of the skin of the nasal vestibule is termed nasal vestibulitis. It may be secondary to constant rhinorrhea, nose picking, or viral infections such as herpes simplex and herpes zoster. Foreign bodies frequently cause vestibulitis in children due to purulent discharge. Nasal furunculosis is *Staphylococcus aureus* infection of the hair follicles. Nose picking is a frequent cause of furunculosis. Topical and if necessary systemic antibiotics are prescribed. The patient should be instructed not to squeeze out pus from this area. Since the veins draining this area are valveless and directly join the cavernous sinus, there is a potential risk of spreading infection to the cavernous sinus via these facial veins. Eczema may also mimic vestibulitis. In these cases steroid base ointment may help the patient. In persistent vestibulitis, neoplastic diseases such as basal cell or squamous cell carcinoma should be kept in mind.

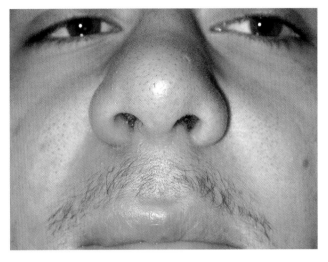

Fig. 2.4.2 If not treated, the infection in the nasal vestibule may spread to the upper lip. The upper lip on the right side appears hyperemic and edematous

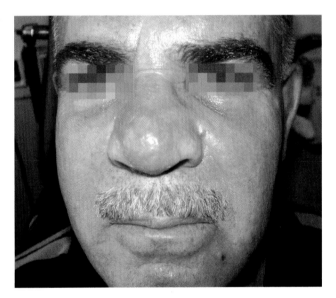

Fig. 2.4.3 Furunculosis in the nasal vestibule with spread of the infection to the nasal tip and dorsum

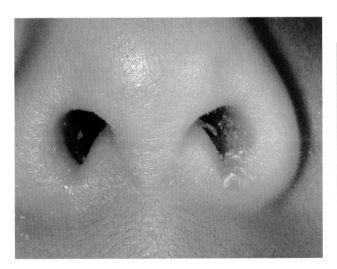

Fig. 2.4.1 Nasal vestibulitis on the left side. Note the slight edema and hyperemia as well as excoriation of the skin on the left side

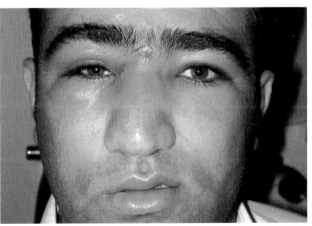

Fig. 2.4.4 Infection starting as nasal vestibulitis with spread of infection to the nasal dorsum and right periorbital area

a

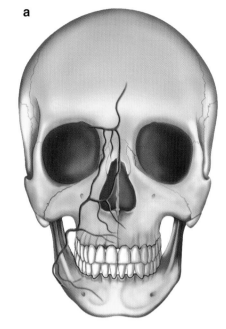

b

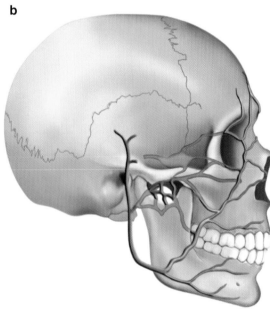

Fig. 2.4.5 Venous drainage of the nose. (**a**) frontal view, (**b**) Lateral view. Since the veins draining this area are valveless and directly join the cavernous sinus, there is a potential risk of spreading infection to the cavernous sinus via these facial veins. This area of the nose is termed the danger triangle. Squeezing the pus from this area should be avoided

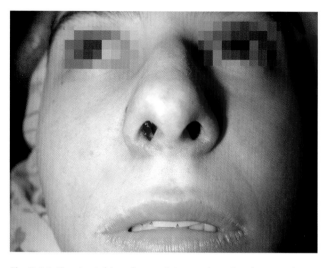

Fig. 2.4.6 Constant rhinorrhea and the need to wipe the nose due to allergic rhinitis have resulted in vestibulitis

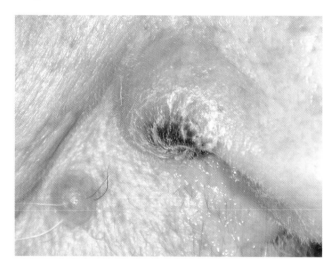

Fig. 2.4.7 Right alar rim. Basal cell carcinoma with slight hyperemia around it. In persistent vestibulitis, neoplastic diseases such as basal cell or squamous cell carcinoma should be kept in mind

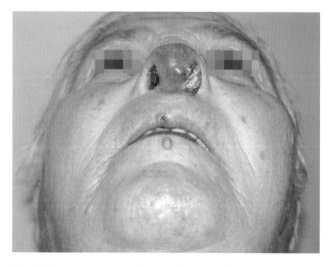

Fig. 2.4.8 Hyperemia and edema in the columella and nasal tip mimicking severe vestibulitis secondary to squamous cell carcinoma infiltration. The neoplastic lesion is filling the left nasal passage

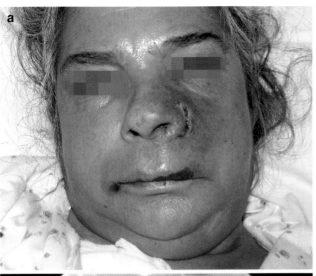

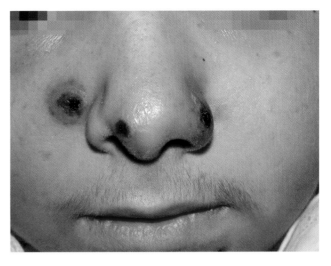

Fig. 2.4.10 Mucormycosis in a child with leukemia. Gross tissue necrosis with a black eschar is characteristic of mucormycosis

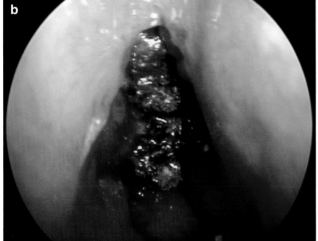

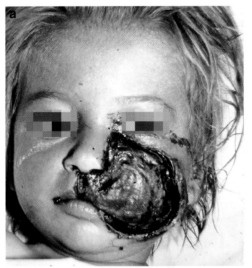

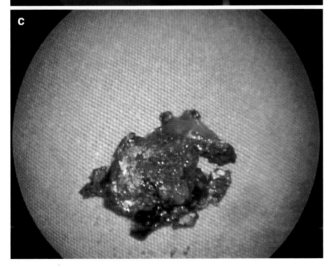

Fig. 2.4.9 Mucormycosis in a diabetic patient. Mucormycosis may infect different areas of the body, but the most frequent fatal form is the rhinocerebral form. (**a**) Necrotic areas on the face, (**b**) black necrotic areas in the nasal mucosa, (**c**) and after removal of necrotic area in the nose

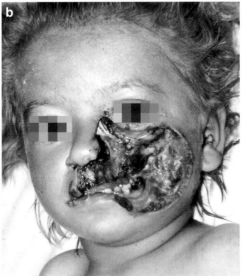

Fig. 2.4.11 (a, b) Mucormycosis in an immunocompromised child. The disease progresses rapidly with extension of tissue necrosis out of the nose into the orbit and face. Local management requires wide debridement of necrotic tissue with a margin of normal-appearing tissue (Courtesy of TESAV)

2.5

Sinusitis

According to the duration of the disease, sinusitis is divided into two categories: acute and chronic.

Acute rhinosinusitis (ARS) is defined as the sudden onset of symptoms lasting less than 12 weeks (with sypmtom free intervals-complete resolution of symptoms, if the problem is recurrent). ARS can occur once or more than once in a defined time period. This is usually expressed as episodes/year, but there must be complete resolution of symptoms between episodes for it to constitute recurrent ARS.

Chronic rhinosinusitis (CRS) is defined as disease lasting more than 12 weeks without complete resolution of symptoms. CRS may also be subject to exacerbations.

The presence of polypoid degeneration in the maxillary sinus deserves special attention. If the polyp is on the floor of the antrum, dental disease should be suspected. If the polyp is on the roof of the antrum, carcinoma should be ruled out in elderly patients. Any evidence of bone erosion should raise the possibility of carcinoma. In patients over 40 years of age, the possibility of carcinoma should always be kept in mind and intrasinus exploration should be performed if necessary.

a

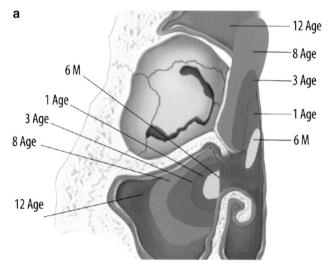

b

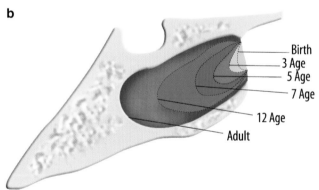

Fig. 2.5.1 Developmental anatomy of the ethmoidal, frontal, and maxillary sinuses (**a**) and sphenoidal sinus (**b**). The ethmoidal and maxillary sinuses are present at birth. The sphenoidal sinus is in the form of a small invagination and develops later. The frontal sinus develops from the anterior ethmoidal cells and moves from an infraorbital position to a supraorbital position, starting to develop at the age of 7. *Yellow*, 6 months; *red*, 1 year; *green*, 3 years; *blue*, 8 years; *maroon*, 12 years of age, adult size

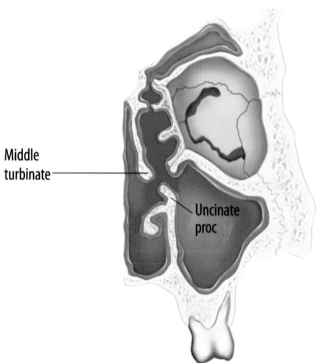

Fig. 2.5.2 Ostiomeatal complex area (OMC) (*blue*). The frontal, maxillary, and anterior ethmoidal cells drain to the OMC. It is a narrow area. Any edema may cause contact of the mucosal surfaces, which may lead to impaired mucociliary activity

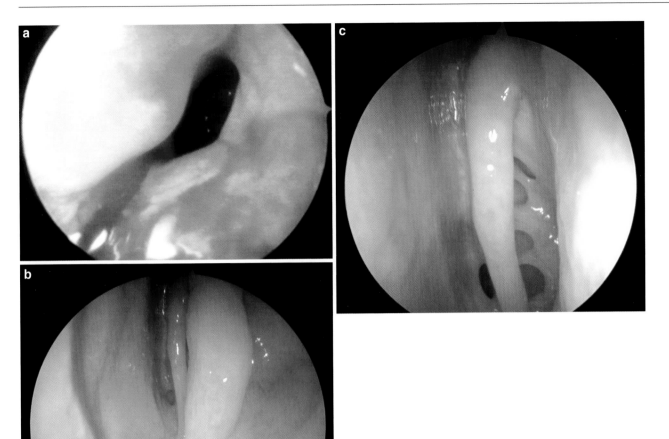

Fig. 2.5.3 (a) Maxillary sinus ostium from nasal side, (b) OMC lateral to the middle turbinate. Superior and posterior to the middle turbinate, the superior turbinate and sphenoid sinus ostium are seen; (c) superior turbinate. Lateral to the superior turbinate are the posterior ethmoidal cells, and medial to the superior turbinate is the sphenoidal sinus ostium

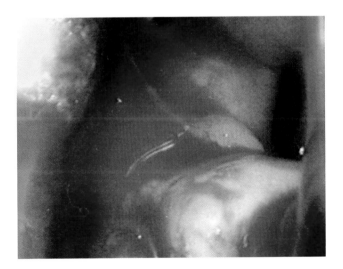

Fig. 2.5.4 Maxillary sinus ostium from the maxillary sinus side. Mucociliary activity is toward the ostium

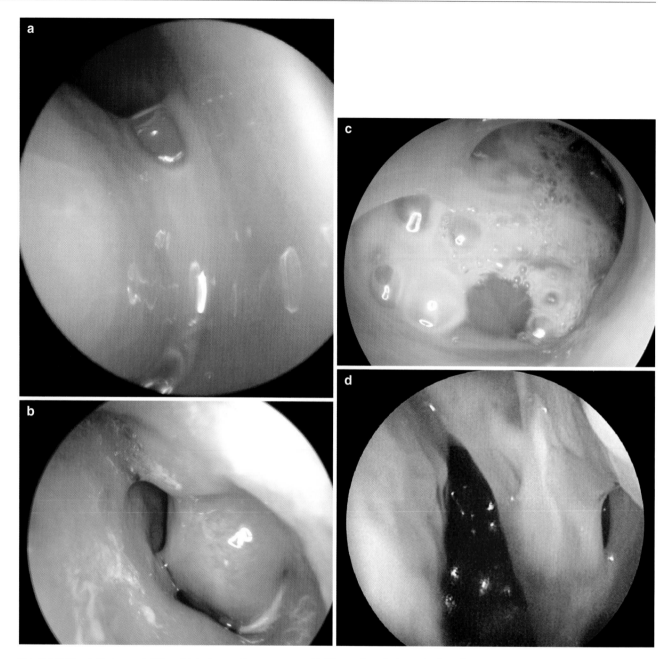

Fig. 2.5.5 Nasal discharge. (**a**) Mucoid drainage after common cold; (**b**) purulent drainage in the inferior meatus; (**c**) postnasal purulent drainage; (**d**) allergic mucin: viscid, thick *yellow–green* drainage, generally eosinophilic

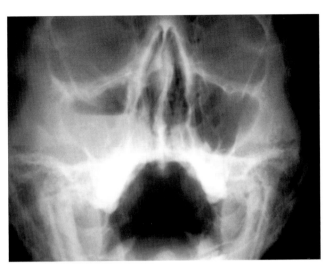

Fig. 2.5.6 Waters view showing right acute maxillary sinusitis. There is an air–fluid level in the right maxillary sinus

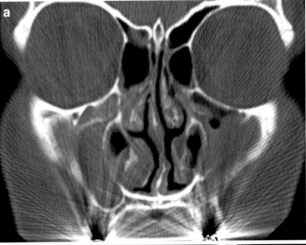

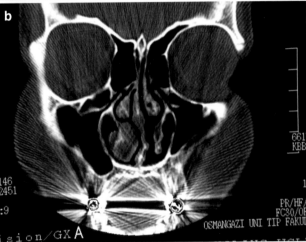

Fig. 2.5.8 (a) Coronal CT shows bilateral maxillary sinusitis; (b) 15 days after starting medical treatment the sinuses appear to be normal

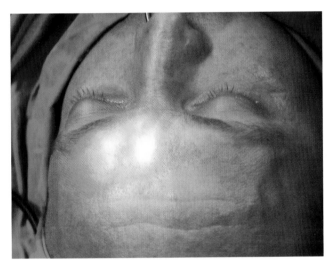

Fig. 2.5.7 Transillumination of the frontal sinus. In frontal sinusitis the frontal sinus fails to transilluminate

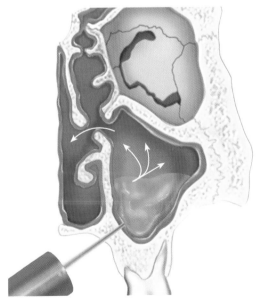

Fig. 2.5.9 Maxillary sinus irrigation. An opening is created via the inferior meatus between the nose and maxillary sinus or via canine fossa

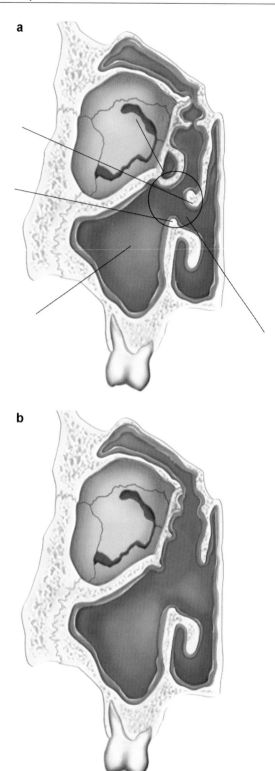

a

b

Fig. 2.5.10 The purpose of endoscopic sinus surgery is to restore ventilation and drainage of the paranasal sinuses. (**a**) Preoperative and (**b**) postoperative view

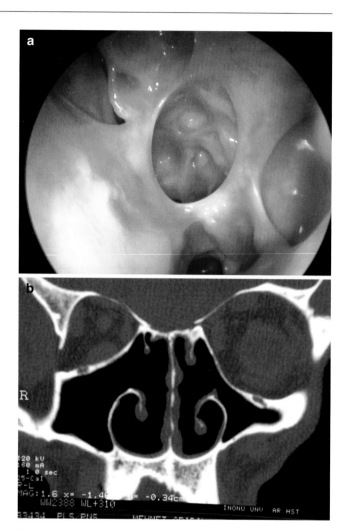

a

b

Fig. 2.5.11 (**a**) Epithelized sinuses and normal mucosa of the sinuses after endoscopic sinus surgery. (**b**) Coronal CT after surgery shows that all sinuses are clean and ostia are open

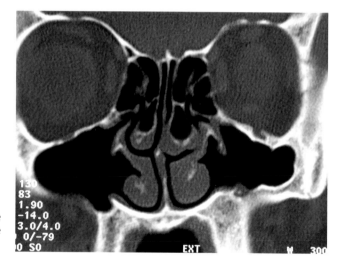

Fig. 2.5.12 Coronal paranasal sinus CT showing previously performed bilateral Caldwell-Luc operation. Note that both nasoantral windows in the inferior meatus are widely open

Fig. 2.5.13 Different areas in the nasal cavity may cause referred pain in various regions of the head

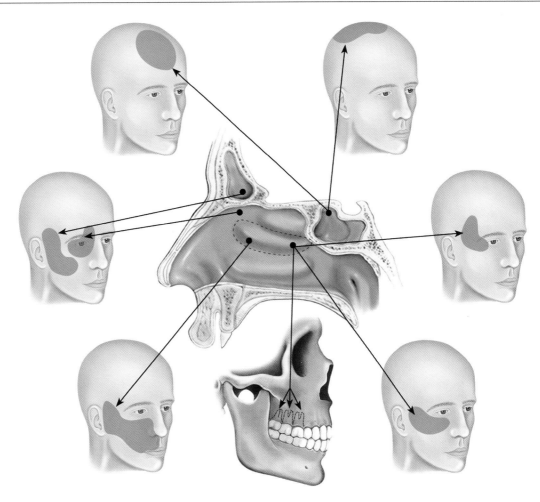

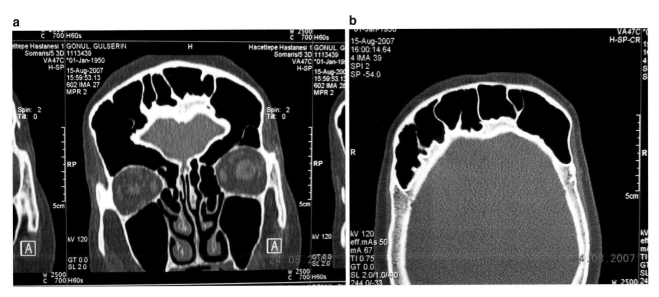

Fig. 2.5.14 (a, b) Overpneumatized frontal sinuses may cause annoying headaches due to negative pressure in the sinus in the frontal area. The pain is generally described as dull

Table 2.5.1 Why is the ostiomeatal complex (OMC) so important in sinusitis?

It is the most commonly diseased site
It is poorly visualized with anterior rhinoscopy
It cannot be evaluated with conventional X-rays
It is a very narrow area, and minor swellings cause obstruction
Symptoms are mild and overshadowed

Table 2.5.2 Sinus aspiration and irrigation indications

Clinical nonresponse to adequate conventional therapy
Immunocompromised patient
Severe symptoms of facial pain
Impending or presenting complications (intraorbital or intracranial)

Table 2.5.3 Sinusitis: host factors

Septal deformity: inhibits drainage of sinuses into the middle meatus
Molar tooth abscess: leads to unilateral maxillary sinusitis
Immunocompromised patients: leukemia – chemotherapy – diabetes – AIDS
Aspirin sensitivity
Intranasal foreign body

Table 2.5.4 Patients who should be referred to ENT surgeon

All frontal or sphenoidal sinuses unresponsive to medical therapy
All immunocompromised patients
All patients with complications of sinus disease
Chronic sinusitis unresponsive to medical management
Chronic sinusitis in children (consider adenoidectomy)

Table 2.5.5 Treatment scheme for primary care for adults with acute rhinosinusitis [Adapted from European Position Paper in Rhinosinusitis and Nasal Polyposis, Suppl 20, 2007]

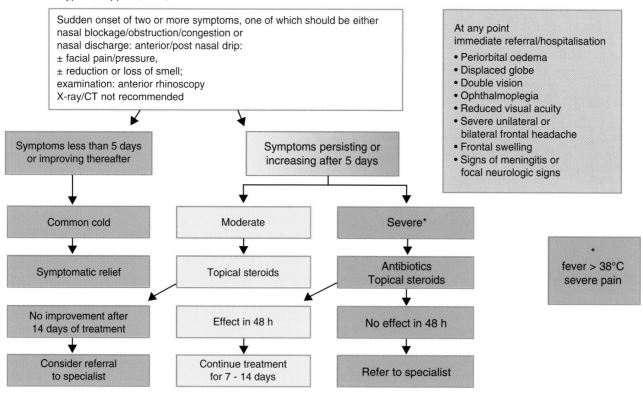

2.6

Complications of Sinusitis

Although the incidence of complications of sinusitis decreased remarkably after the introduction of antibiotics, these complications may still be life threatening. Complications of sinusitis can be classified as local, orbital, and intracranial.

The most popular example of a local complication is frontal bone osteomyelitis. Frontal sinusitis may cause osteomyelitis of the anterior table of the frontal bone. The pus may collect between the bone and periosteum. This subperiosteal abscess is known as "Pott's puffy tumor." Orbital complications are very frequently due to ethmoidal sinusitis. Especially in children, the lamina papyracea is dehiscent and infection can easily spread to the orbit.

Table 2.6.1 Complications of sinusitis

Osteomyelitis
Frontal (Pott's puffy tumor)
Intracranial
Epidural abscess
Subdural abscess
Cavernous sinus thrombosis
Meningitis
Brain abscess
Orbital
Inflammatory edema (periorbital cellulitis)
Subperiosteal abscess
Orbital cellulitis
Orbital abscess
Optic neuritis (cavernous sinus thrombophlebitis)

Table 2.6.2 Extension routes of infection in sinusitis[a]

Osteitis (osteomyelitis in bones with bone marrow)
Direct extension
Congenital dehiscences
Fracture lines from previous head traumas
Venous extension
Retrograde thrombophlebitis between the sinus mucosal veins and orbital and dural veins; Septic emboli in diploic veins[b]

[a]Lymphatic spread plays no role in extension of sinus infections
[b]There are no valves in the veins connecting the orbit and sinuses (Breschet diploic veins) and this creates an easy route for extension of infection

Table 2.6.3 Stages of orbital complications of sinusitis

Periorbital cellulitis	Infection anterior to the orbital septum
Orbital cellulitis	Infection posterior to the orbital septum
Subperiosteal abscess	Pus collection beneath the periosteum and lamina papyracea
Orbital abscess	Pus collection in the orbit
Cavernous sinus thrombophlebitis	Extension of infection to cavernous sinus

Table 2.6.4 Orbital complications, eye mobility vs. vision

Complication	Extraocular muscle impairment	Visual acuity loss
Inflammatory edema	None	None
Subperiosteal abscess	Minimal, in early stages; may limit eye mobility significantly in big abscesses	None, very minimal in big abscesses
Orbital cellulitis	Minimal	Minimal
Orbital abscess	Complete	Severe
Cavernous sinus thrombosis	Complete, often bilateral	Severe, often bilateral

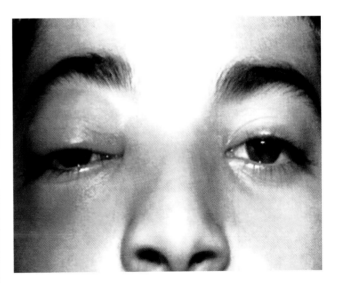

Fig. 2.6.1 Right preseptal cellulitis. It is seen particularly in children because of the dehiscences in the lamina papyracea. Sometimes when the ethmoid sinus is completely congested, periorbital swelling may occur due to obstruction of venous drainage

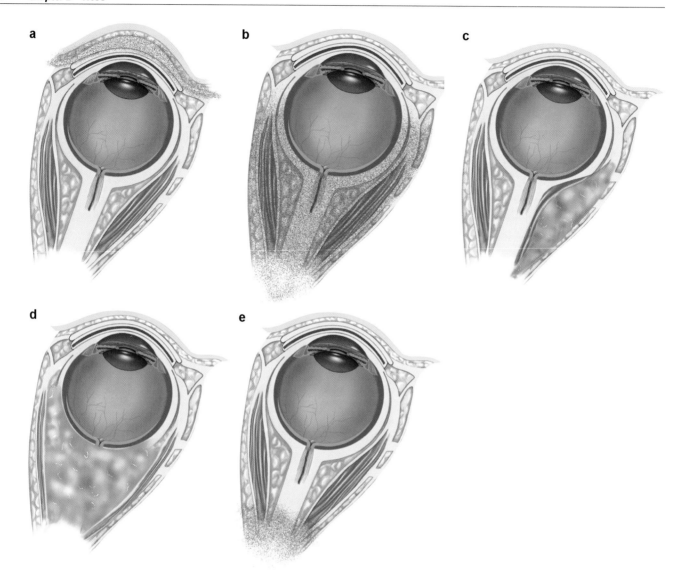

Fig. 2.6.2 Schematic drawing of orbital complications of sinusitis. (**a**) Preseptal cellulitis, (**b**) orbital cellulitis, (**c**) subperiosteal abscess, (**d**) orbital abscess, and (**e**) cavernous sinus thrombophlebitis

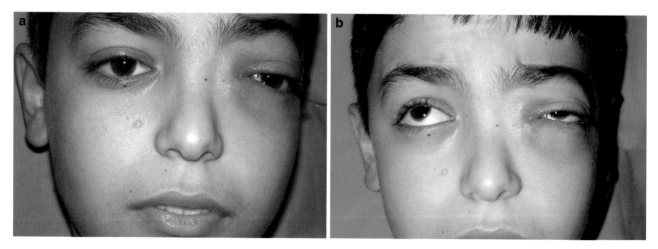

Fig. 2.6.3 Left-sided subperiosteal abscess. (**a**) The eye globe is pushed anteriorly and is displaced laterally and inferiorly by the subperiosteal abscess. The patient's upper lid is swollen, and (**b**) he is unable to elevate his left upper eyelid. His eye movements are limited in the upward and medial gaze. (**c**) Axial CT scan shows com- plete opacification of the left ethmoid cells. There is a large subperiosteal abscess lateral to the lamina papyracea. Very small bony dehiscences can be noted in the lamina papyracea; (**d**) axial and (**e**) coronal MR images demonstrate complete opacification of ethmoid sinuses and large subperiosteal abscess

c

d

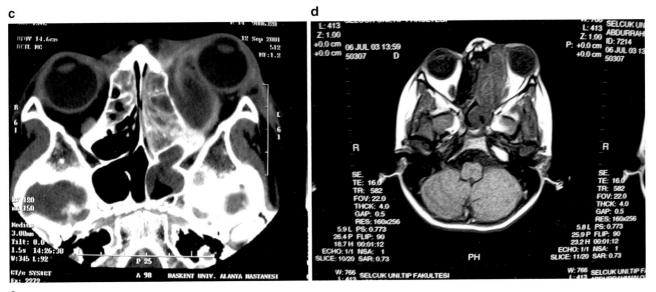

e

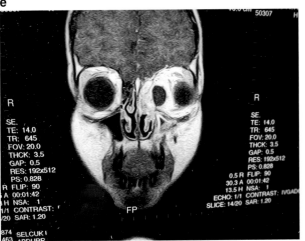

Fig. 2.6.3 (continued)

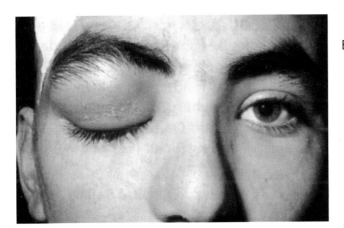

Fig. 2.6.4 Right orbital abscess due to ethmoiditis. Infection from the ethmoid sinuses may spread very easily via small dehiscences in the lamina papyracea into the orbit. External drainage may be required

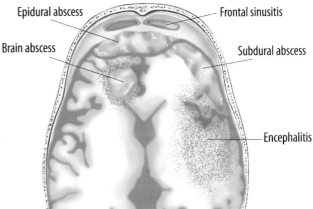

Fig. 2.6.5 Schematic representation of intracranial complications of frontal sinusitis. Purulent material may collect between the bone and dura (epidural abscess) or between the dura and the brain (subdural abscess) or in the brain (brain abscess)

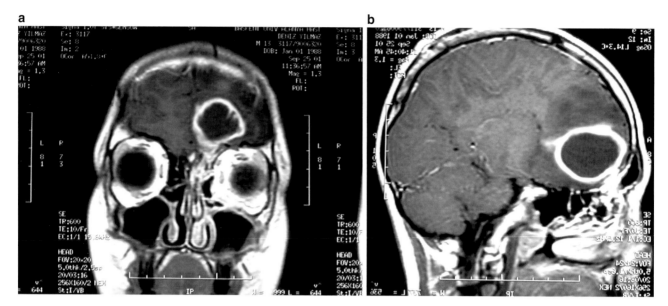

Fig. 2.6.6 Brain abscess. (**a**) Coronal and (**b**) sagittal MR images

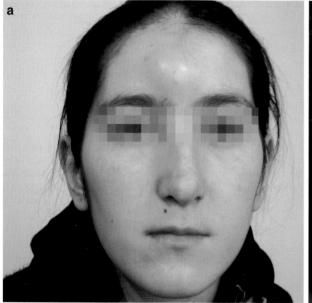
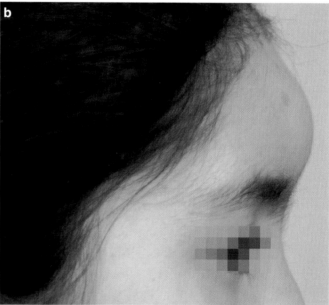

Fig. 2.6.7 Pott's puffy tumor. Following acute frontal sinusitis, the patient developed subperiosteal abscess in the forehead area. The forehead is swollen, tender, and fluctuant. (**a**) Frontal view, (**b**) lateral view, (**c, d**) axial MR images, (**e**) and sagittal reconstruction (the frontal sinus is opaque). Subperiosteal abscess is seen under the soft tissues of the forehead

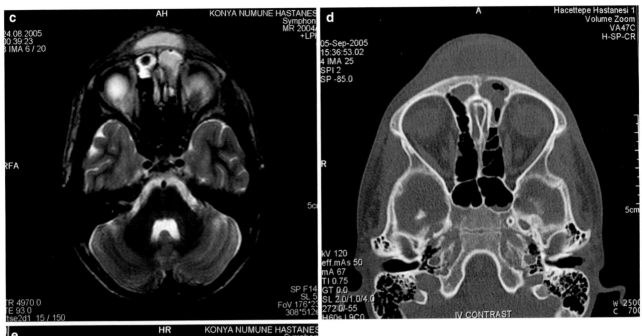

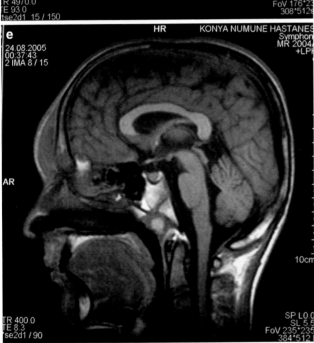

Fig. 2.6.7 (continued)

Fig. 2.6.8 (a, b) Axial and coronal CT scans of frontal sinus mucocele. The ethmoid sinuses are completely opaque, and the posterior and superior wall of the frontal sinus is destroyed. Erosion of the roof of the orbit leads to orbital displacement inferiorly and laterally

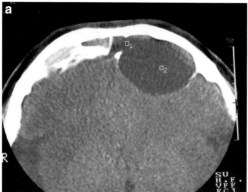
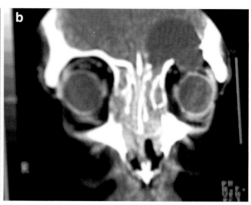

Fig. 2.6.9 Left-sided ophthalmoplegia. The eye globe does not move in any direction. **(a)** The left upper lid is ptotic; **(b)** left eye does not move in lateral direction; **(c)** left eye does not move in medial direction; **(d)** left eye does not move in inferior direction; **(e)** left eye does not move in superior direction. Superior orbital fissure syndrome is characterized by the involvement of the 3rd, 4th, 6th, and ophthalmic branch of the trigeminal nerve. Vision is normal. In orbital apex syndrome, the optic foramen is also involved and there is loss of vision due to optic nerve involvement in addition to the superior orbital fissure syndrome

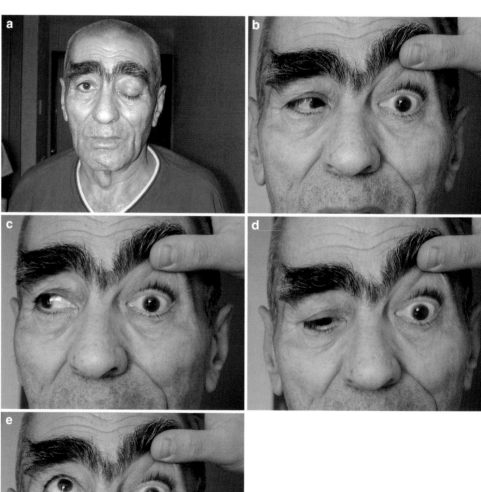
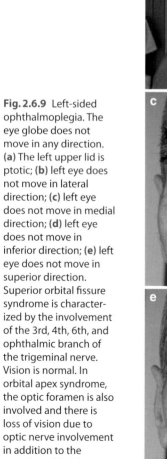

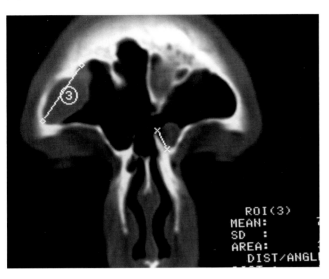

Fig. 2.6.10 Supraorbital frontal cell in the lateral wall of the frontal sinus. If they do not cause any symptoms, there is no need for surgery. To treat these disorders, osteoplastic frontal sinus operation is necessary

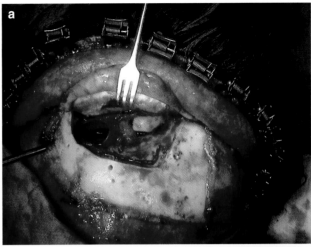

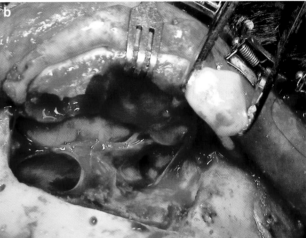

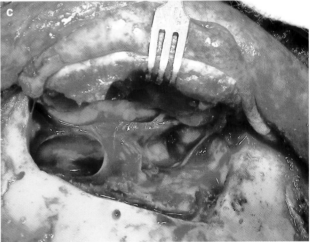

Fig. 2.6.11 (a–c) Osteoplastic frontal sinus operation in a patient with frontal sinus osteoma. The anterior table of the frontal sinus is elevated. The periosteum is not separated from the anterior table and is pedicled on the bone. After removing the osteoma and cleaning the pathology, the anterior table is placed back into the original position. Although this procedure is performed rarely, it provides a wide exposure in complicated diseases, trauma, tumor, or CSF fistula of the frontal sinus

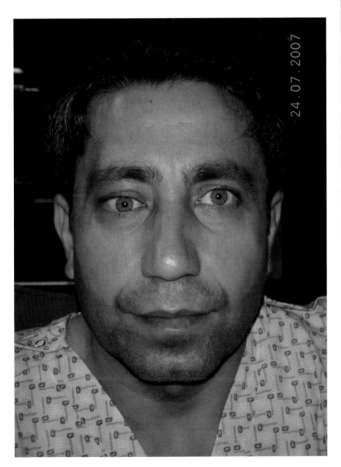

Fig. 2.6.12 Due to ethmoidofrontal mucocele, the right eye is pushed laterally and inferiorly. The eye globes are not at the same level

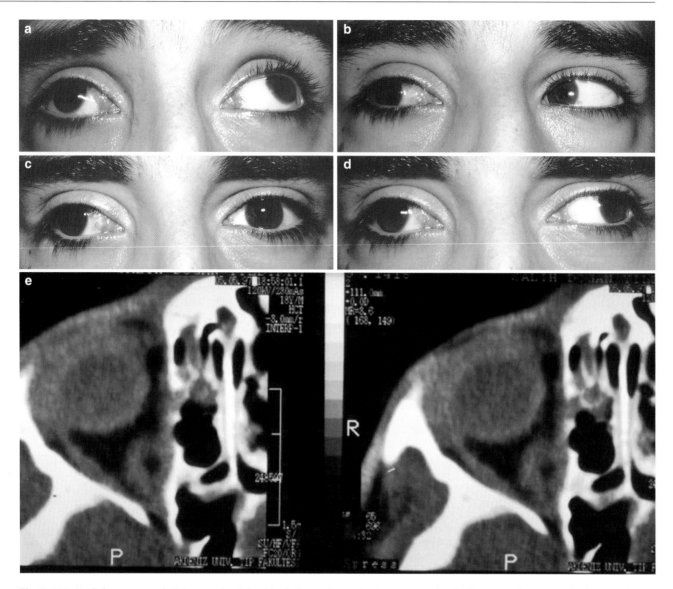

Fig. 2.6.13 Medial rectus muscle injury on the right side during endoscopic sinus surgery. (**a–d**) There is strabismus to the lateral side and impaired mobility of the eye. (**e**) Axial CT scans show the injury (courtesy of Şener)

2.7

Nasal Polyposis

Polyps are one of the most frequent causes of nasal obstruction. Polyps may be isolated or diffuse. The behavior of nasal polyps depends on the type of granulocytes. Eosinophils play a significant role in the classification of polyps. Polyps with significant eosinophilia behave differently from those with neutrophils. The majority of diffuse nasal polyposis is eosinophilic. Analgesic intolerance and asthma might accompany diffuse eosinophilic nasal polyposis in the later decades of a patient's life. Isolated polyps can originate from an anatomic structure such as the ethmoid bulla or uncinate process. If polyps originate from the mucosa inside the sinus, they are named according to the sinus. If the polyp originates from the maxillary sinus it is called an antrochoanal polyp, and if it originates from the sphenoid sinus it is called a sphenochoanal polyp.

Nasal polyps are unusual in children. If a child presents with nasal polyposis, the possibility of diseases such as cystic fibrosis or primary ciliary dyskinesia should be eliminated. If the nasal polyp is unilateral, nasal encephaloceles should be ruled out with MR imaging.

In diffuse nasal polyposis patients, the presence of asthma or analgesic intolerance should always be questioned. Due to the danger of intolerance which can develop later in their life, NSAIDs should not be prescribed to patients with diffuse eosinophilic nasal polyposis.

In adults, unilateral polyps should always raise the clinical suspicion of malignancy.

Table 2.7.1 Classification of nasal polyposis

Polyps
Inflammatory
Choanal/ isolated
Eosinophilic
Additional criteria
Acetylsalicylic acid intolerance
Asthma/COPD
Allergy
Associated diseases
Cystic fibrosis
Immune insufficiency (acquired/congenital)
Primary ciliary dyskinesia
Vasculitis, granulomatosis

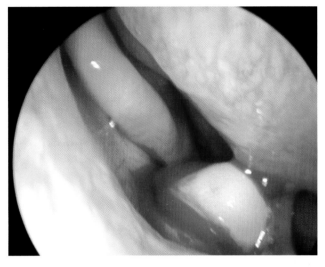

Fig. 2.7.1 Isolated polyp originating from the right middle meatus and extending anterior to the middle turbinate

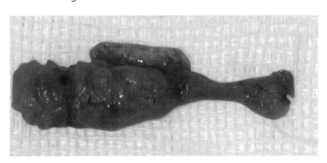

Fig. 2.7.2 Polyp originating from the uncinate process

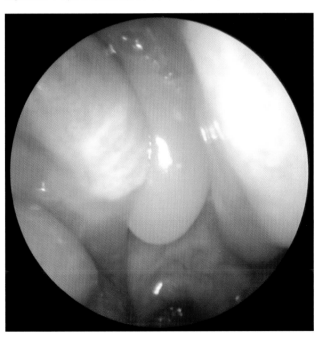

Fig. 2.7.3 Right sphenochoanal polyp originating from the mucosa inside the sphenoid sinus, filling the sphenoethmoidal recess, and extending to the choana

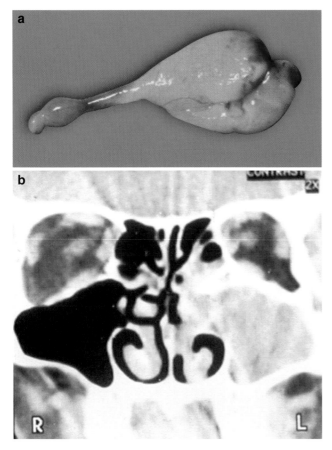

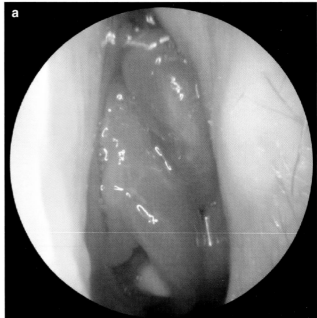

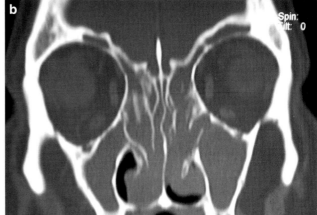

Fig. 2.7.4 (a) Antrochoanal polyp has three parts. The cystic portion is the part originating in the maxillary sinus. If this part is not removed, the polyp recurs. The neck is the portion of the polyp passing through the ostium. The main polyp mass is the part filling the nasal passage and causing obstruction. Although antrochoanal polyps are very often unilateral, they may cause bilateral nasal obstruction by extending and occluding the other choana. If the cystic part is not removed, the polyp recurs. **(b)** Coronal CT scan of antrochoanal polyp; the left maxillary sinus is opaque and the maxillary sinus ostium is widened. This widening of the maxillary sinus ostium is almost diagnostic for antrochoanal polyp

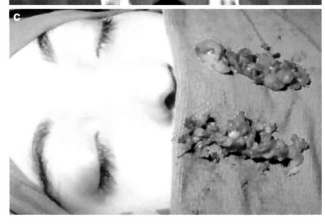

Fig. 2.7.5 (a) Diffuse eosinophilic nasal polyposis; the nasal passage is completely obstructed. Since the whole ethmoidal mucosa is polypoid there is no originating point. **(b)** Coronal CT scan shows that all sinuses are opaque. **(c)** Removal of the polyps

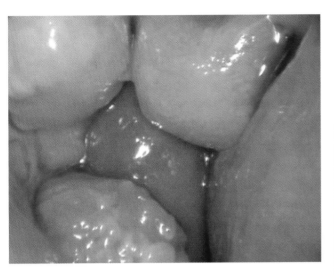

Fig. 2.7.6 Diffuse eosinophilic nasal polyposis completely obstructing the nasal passage

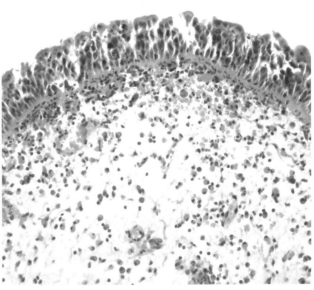

Fig. 2.7.8 Diffuse nasal polyposis. Diffuse eosinophilia is seen on histological examination (H&E)

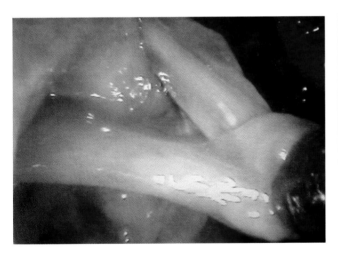

Fig. 2.7.7 In eosinophilic diffuse nasal polyposis, the mucus is thick, viscid, and *yellow-green*. It contains many eosinophils. It is referred to as allergic mucin

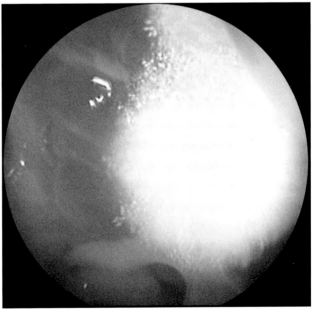

Fig. 2.7.9 Fungal ball in sphenoid sinus

EAR

NOSE

THROAT AND NECK

a

b

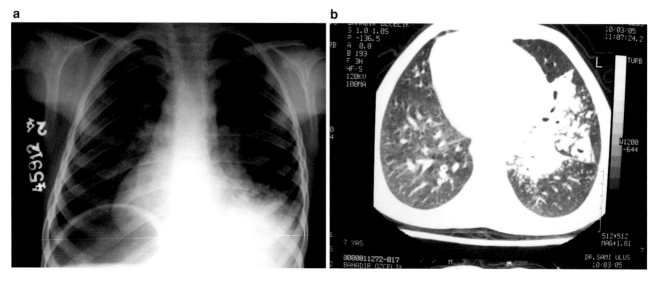

Fig. 2.7.10 Kartagener syndrome. (**a**) Dextrocardia on chest X-ray; (**b**) diffuse bronchiectasia on axial CT scan

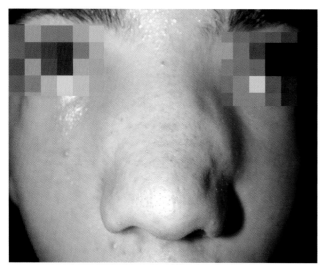

Fig. 2.7.11 Nasal bone expansion due to extensive diffuse nasal polyposis in the younger patient. Rhinoplasty is needed to restore the appearance

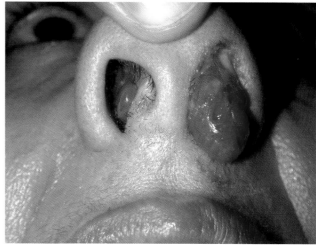

Fig. 2.7.12 Diffuse nasal polyposis completely filling the nasal passages. On the left side, nasal polyps protrude from the nostril. The patient did not agree to the operation because of her fear of anesthesia

Table 2.7.2 Treatment evidence and recommendations for postoperative treatment in adults with nasal polyps[a]

Therapy	Level	Grade of recommendation	Relevance
Oral antibiotics: short term < 2 weeks	No data	D	Immediately postoperative, if pus was seen during operation
Oral antibiotics: long term > 12 weeks	Ib	A	Yes
Topical steroids after Functional endoscopic sinus surgery (FESS)	Ib (two studies one +, one −)	B	Yes
Topical steroids after polypectomy	Ib	A	Yes
Oral steroids	No data	D	Yes
Nasal douche	No data	D	Yes

After Table 13.6 of European Position Paper in Rhinosinusitis and Nasal Polyposis, Suppl 20, 2007. Reproduced with permission of *Rhinology*
[a]Some of these studies also included patients with Chronic Rhinosinusitis (CRS) without nasal polyps

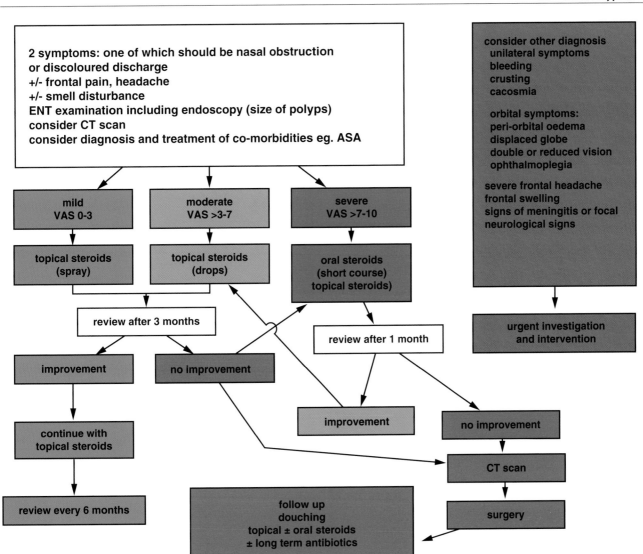

Table. 2.7.3 Treatment scheme for ENT specialists for adults with nasal polyps. After Fig. 13.5 of European Position Paper in Rhinosinusitis and Nasal Polyposis, Suppl 20, 2007. Reproduced with permission of *Rhinology*

2.8

Nasal Obstruction

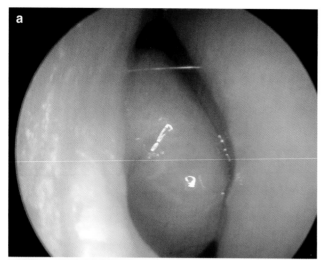

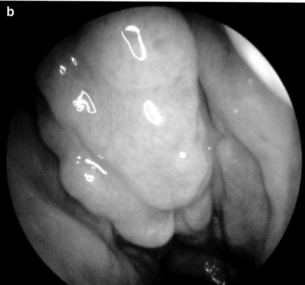

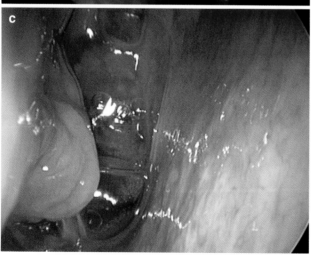

Fig. 2.8.1 **(a)** Right inferior turbinate hypertrophy. **(b)** Nodular type left inferior turbinate hypertrophy. **(c)** Posterior part of the inferior turbinate is polypoid causing nasal obstruction

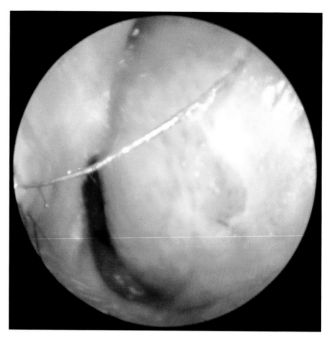

Fig. 2.8.2 Septal deviation to the right

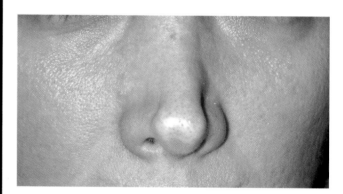

Fig. 2.8.3 Nasal obstruction due to alar insufficiency, which is the result of overexcision of the lateral crura of the lower lateral cartilages during rhinoplasty. The depressions on both sides lateral to the nasal tip are due to overresection of the alar cartilages

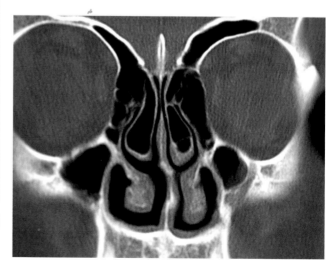

Fig. 2.8.4 Bilateral concha bullosa. No surgery is necessary for asymptomatic cases

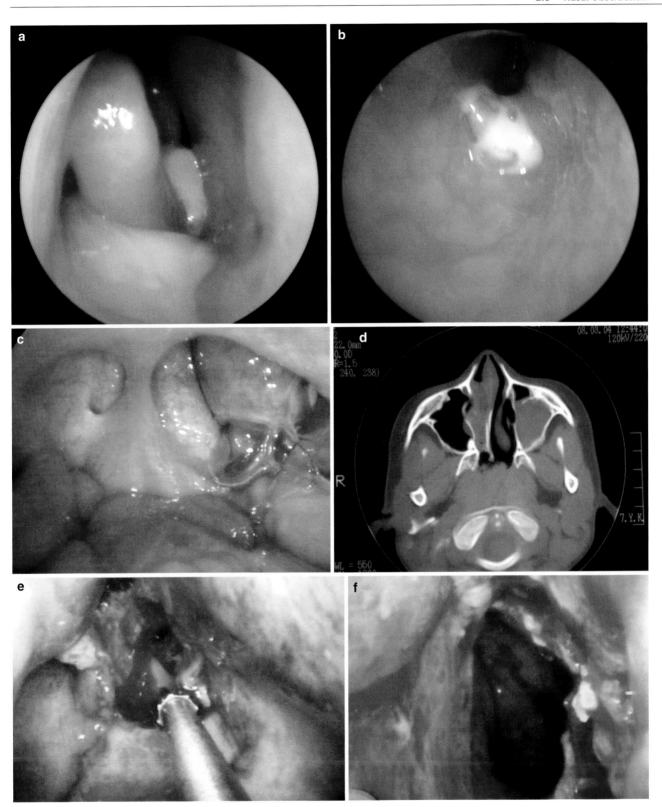

Fig. 2.8.5 Choanal atresia is a congenital abnormality. A bony plate or a membrane obstructs the posterior nares. Unilateral atresia may not cause symptoms. However, bilateral choanal atresia presents an emergency situation since the newborn is totally dependent on the nasal airway for breathing. During feeding, the newborn becomes cyanotic. The diagnosis is made by the inability to pass a soft catheter perinasally, or demonstrating the atretic plate after instillation of radiopaque dye. CT scan shows the atretic plate. The atretic plate can be seen on endoscopic examination. As soon as the diagnosis is made, a transnasal airway should be established. Blindly perforating the bony plate or the membrane should be avoided because of the narrow nasopharynx and unsatisfactory results. Endoscopic transnasal surgery of choanal atresia gives better results. (**a**) Mucoid discharge in the nasal cavity. (**b**) Endoscopic view of atretic plate from inside the nose. (**c**) Right-sided unilateral choanal atresia; view from the nasopharynx. (**d**) Axial CT scan shows right-sided unilateral choanal atresia. Note the narrow nasal cavity on the atresia side due to thickened pterygoid plates. (**e**) Mucosal flaps have been elevated and the bony plate is drilled. (**f**) Complete opening of the atresia; the flaps are placed in position, the nasopharynx is seen

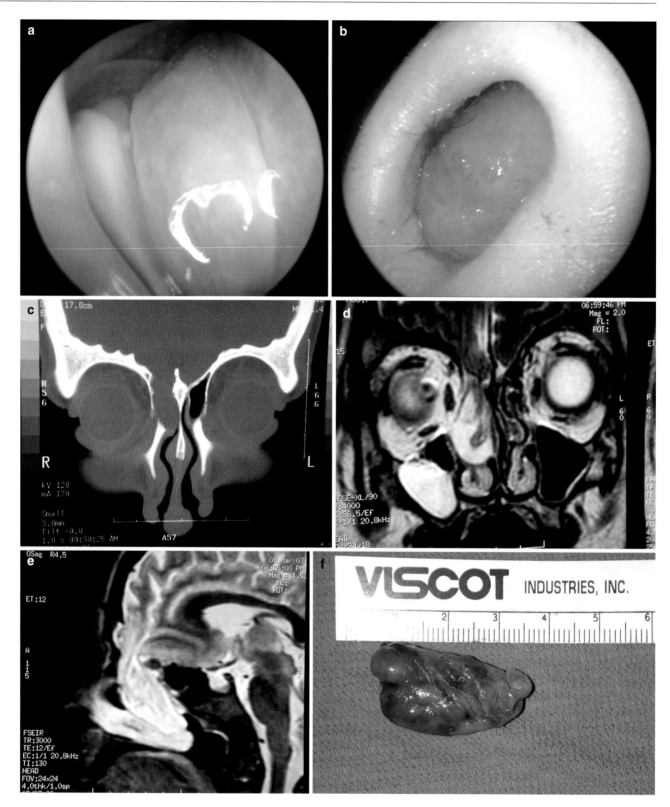

Fig. 2.8.6 Nasal encephaloceles are rare lesions. The brain and meninges herniate through a defect generally in the lamina cribrosa. Encephaloceles are bluish, pulsatile, compressible masses. CT and MR imaging is necessary. Treatment comprises surgical removal of the encephalocele and closure of the defect. (**a, b**) Nasal view of encephaloceles. (**c**) On the coronal CT scan, the defect at the ethmoid roof is visible. (**d, e**) Coronal and sagittal MR images of the encephalocele herniating through the cranial defect into the nasal cavity. (**f**) Encephalocele after resection. (**g**) Closure of the defect with temporalis fascia

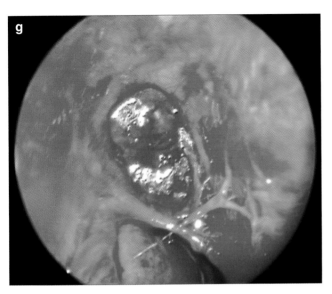

g

Fig. 2.8.6 (Continued)

Table 2.8.1 Nasal obstructions

Rhinitis (acute, chronic)
Mechanical factors
Nasopharyngeal diseases (Thornwald cyst, adenoid vegetation)
Turbinate pathologies
Middle turbinate pathologies (paradox middle turbinate, concha bullosa)
Inferior turbinate hypertrophy
Anatomic abnormalities
Septal deviation, septal abscess
Alar collapse
Nasal valve insufficiency
Choanal atresia
Foreign bodies
Nasal masses
Nasal polyps
Encephalocele
Benign tumors
Malignant tumors

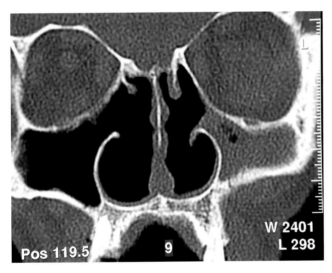

Fig. 2.8.7   Empty nose. Although bilateral functional endoscopic sinus surgery and total inferior turbinate resection were performed in a previous operation, the patient felt that his nose was still obstructed

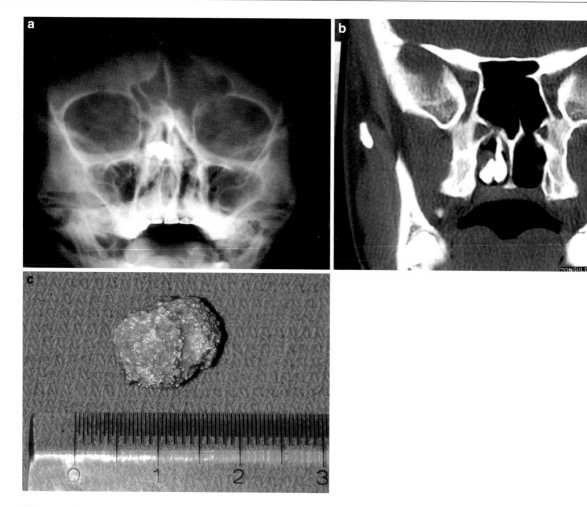

Fig. 2.8.8 Rhinolith. A rhinolith is a large foreign body with deposits of Ca and Mg around a nidus. On examination there is a unilateral mass that is hard on palpation. Radiologic examination helps to make the diagnosis. (**a**) Waters view; an opaque foreign body lateral to the middle turbinate. (**b**) Coronal paranasal sinus CT showing opaque foreign material inferior and lateral to the inferior turbinate. (**c**) The rhinolith after removal

2.9

Septum

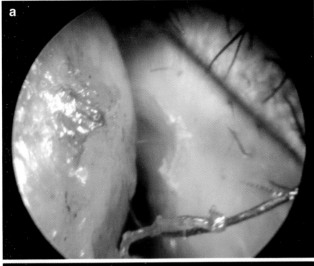

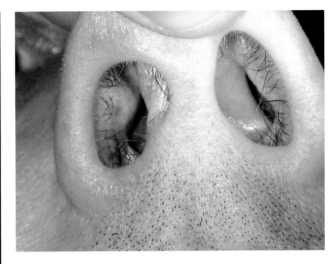

Fig. 2.9.2 Septal spur at the anterior septal area completely obstructing the airway

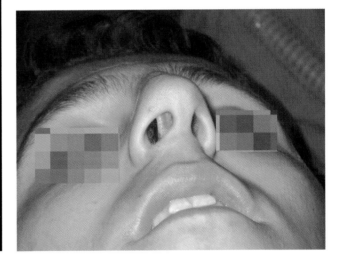

Fig. 2.9.1 **(a)** Septal deviation to the left side. **(b)** Compensatory inferior turbinate hypertrophy on the opposite side

Fig. 2.9.3 Severe caudal dislocation of the septum to the right

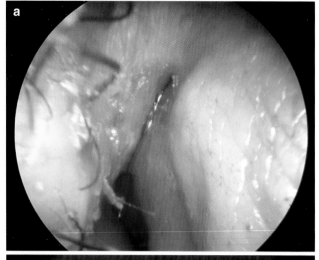

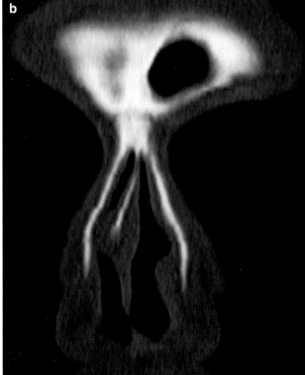

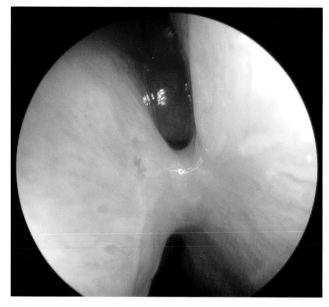

Fig. 2.9.5 Synechia between septum and inferior turbinate

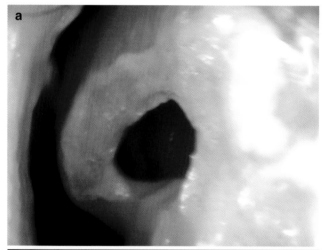

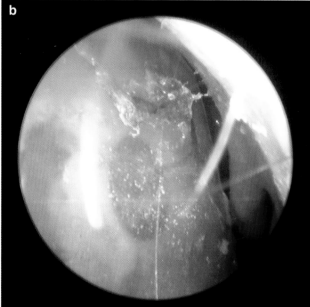

Fig. 2.9.4 **(a)** Septal deviation to the right, which narrows nasal valve area. **(b)** Coronal CT shows narrowing of the nasal valve area

Fig. 2.9.6 Septal perforation. There are many causes of septal perforation. The most common cause is previous septal surgery. Other causes include chronic trauma such as nose-picking, use of cocaine, septal hematomas, and infections like tuberculosis. The majority of perforations are located in the anterior cartilaginous portion of the septum. However, syphilitic infection involves the posterior bony septum. In small perforations a whistling sound may be heard during inspiration. Crusting may cause obstruction. As the crusts break off, bleeding occurs. Steam inhalations, nasal douching, and softening ointments may decrease the crusting. **(a)** Septal perforation after submucous resection. **(b)** Septal button to close the perforation temporarily. Small and medium-sized perforations can be closed by surgery. For bigger perforations, a silastic nasal septal button can be used for occlusion

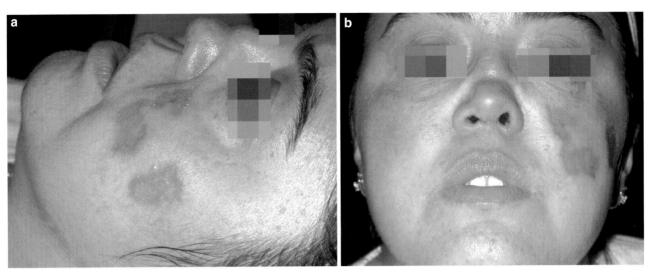

Fig. 2.9.7 **(a, b)** Saddle nose deformity. This was due to dorsal collapse of the nose as a result of cartilage destruction in a patient with tuberculosis

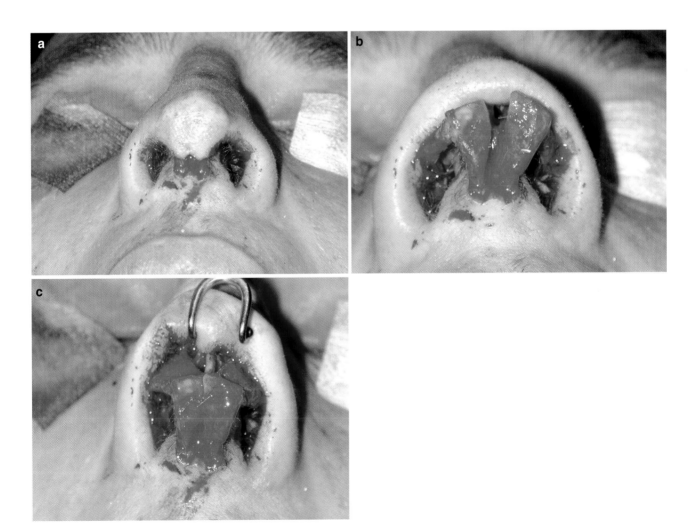

Fig. 2.9.8 External rhinoplasty. **(a)** A transverse incision across the columella, **(b)** elevation of the nasal skin superiorly. **(c)** Suturing lower lateral cartilages

Fig. 2.9.9 (a) Cartilage and bony hump removal. **(b)** To rotate the nasal tip superiorly, the septal cartilage, lower and upper lateral cartilages may be shortened. **(c)** Medial and lateral osteotomies to narrow the nose

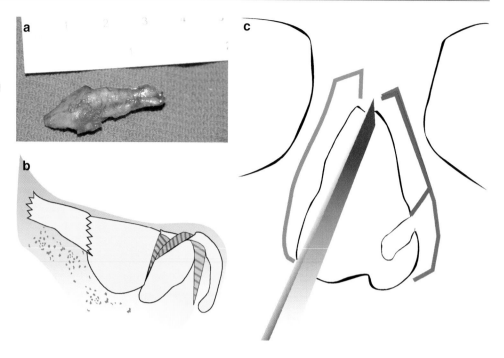

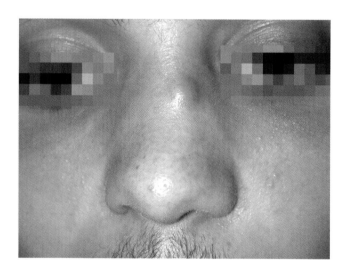

Fig. 2.9.10 Infected cartilage graft at the nasal dorsum after rhinoplasty

2.10

Epistaxis

Although the majority of cases of epistaxis are self-limiting, it may sometimes be very severe and very difficult to manage. In Table 2.10.1, local and systemic factors that may cause epistaxis are presented.

Epistaxis may be from the anterior or posterior septum or nasal cavity. Posterior epistaxis is usually from the sphenopalatine artery and sometimes may be difficult to control and manage. Bleeding from Little's area may be cauterized by silver nitrate.

The patient sits in the upright position. The head should be kept straight and should not be extended in order to keep the intracranial pressure low. The nose should be cleared of clots by blowing. Cotton wool pledgets soaked in appropriate solution are placed in the nasal cavity. In hypertensive patients, adrenaline should not be used. These pledgets show whether the bleeding is from the anterior or posterior side. If the bleeding is from Little's area, it can be cauterized. Anterior packing should be placed in layers. If the epistaxis is from the posterior septal area, then posterior packing may be necessary. Systemic diseases should be treated.

Table 2.10.1 Etiology of epistaxis

Local
Trauma
Inflammation
Postoperative
Foreign body
Nasal and paranasal sinus tumors
Hereditary hemorrhagic telangiectasia
Atrophic rhinitis
Systemic
Hypertension
High venous pressure (mitral stenosis)
Blood dyscrasias (leukemia, hemophilia, vitamin K deficiency)
Anticoagulant drugs

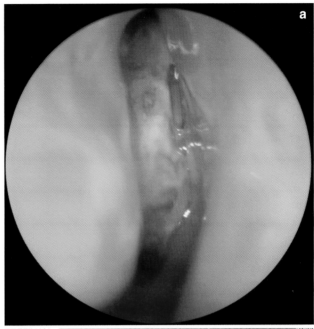
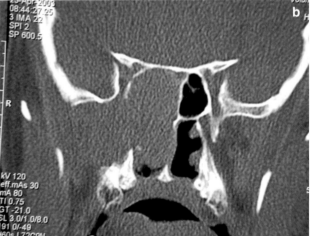
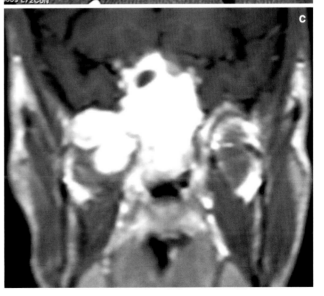

Fig. 2.10.1 Unilateral bleeding and nasal obstruction in a young male patient should raise the suspicion of juvenile nasopharyngeal angiofibroma (JNA). (**a**) Endoscopic view of the JNA in the nose. (**b**) Coronal CT shows widening of the pterygomaxillary fissure. (**c**) Hypervascularity of the tumor

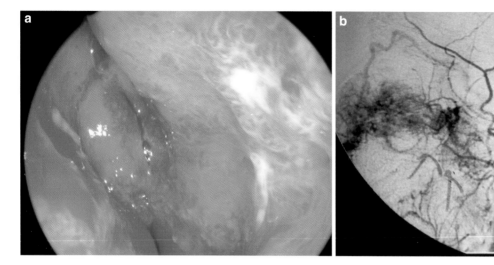

Fig. 2.10.2 (**a**) Hereditary hemorrhagic telangiectasia (Osler-Weber-Rendu disease) is characterized by small abnormal capillaries in the nasal mucosa. It may cause serious nasal bleeding, and hemoglobin levels may drop to very low levels, necessitating blood transfusion. In the nasal mucosa, numerous leashes of bleeding vessels can be seen. Laser coagulation may be effective in the early stages. In severe cases, skin grafting may be necessary. (**b**) Angiography shows hypervascularization

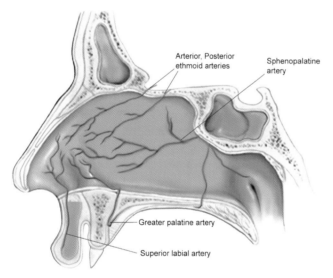

Fig. 2.10.3 Kiesselbach's plexus (Little's area). It is localized at the anterior portion of the septum. Approximately 90% of bleeding occurs from this area. The external and carotid artery systems anastomose in this area. The anterior and posterior ethmoid arteries from the internal carotid artery system and the superior labial artery, greater palatine artery, and sphenopalatine artery from the external carotid artery system form a vascular plexus

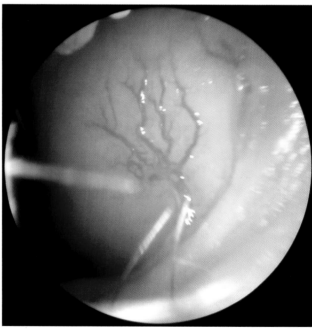

Fig. 2.10.4 Bleeding vessels in Kiesselbach's plexus (Little's area)

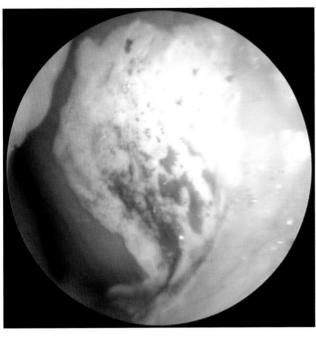

Fig. 2.10.5 Cauterization of Little's area with silver nitrate sticks

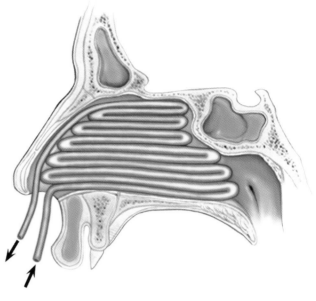

Fig. 2.10.6 Anterior nasal packing with Vaseline-impregnated gauze. After cleaning the clots, the packing is done in layers

Fig. 2.10.7 Posterior nasal packing. A postnasal pack is prepared from a tightly compressed ball of gauze according to the size of the postnasal space and tied with 0-silk ties. A soft rubber catheter is passed along the floor of the nose to the pharynx and taken out through the mouth. One end of the silk tie is attached to the tip of the catheter and drawn back through the nose. The pack is pushed behind the soft palate in the nasopharynx by exerting moderate pressure. The ends of the silk ties are attached near the nose and mouth corner. All patients with posterior nasal packing should be hospitalized for close observation

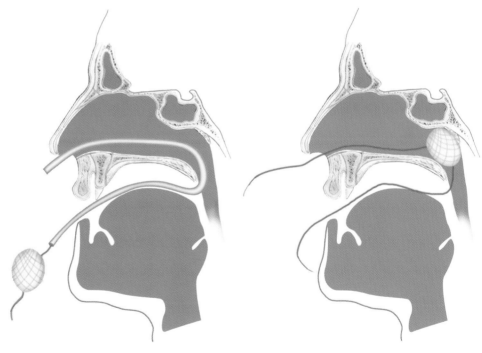

2.11

Traumas

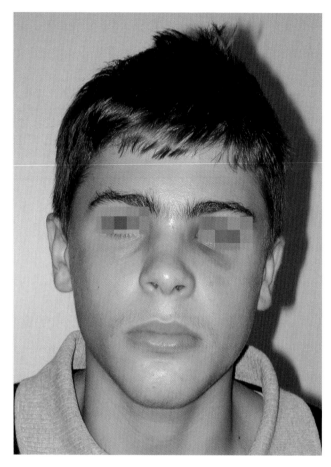

Fig. 2.11.1 Nasal fracture. A blow coming from the lateral side caused the nose to be displaced to the other side. There is ecchymosis in the infraorbital area

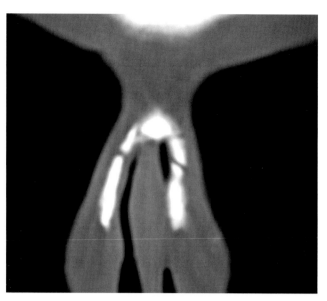

Fig. 2.11.3 Coronal CT scan showing multiple fractures of the nasal bones

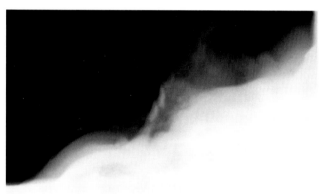

Fig. 2.11.4 Lateral X-ray showing nasal bone fracture. Depression of the nasal bones requires the elevation of the depressed bony fragments

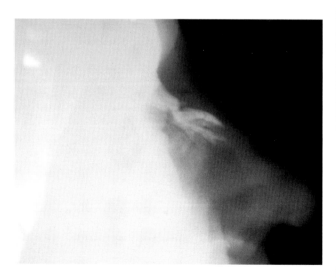

Fig. 2.11.2 Lateral X-ray. Nasal fracture shows displacement of nasal bones

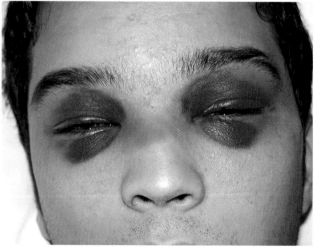

Fig. 2.11.5 Raccoon eyes or periorbital ecchymosis is a sign of basal skull fracture. It results from blood from the skull fracture tracking down into the soft tissue around the eyes (courtesy of Dr. Kıratlı)

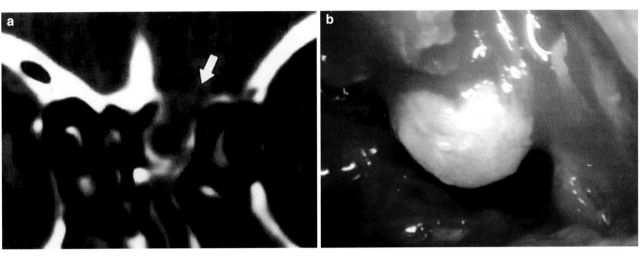

Fig. 2.11.6 Cerebrospinal fluid rhinorrhea after trauma. (**a**) Coronal CT showing herniation through the lamina cribrosa at the anterior ethmoid area. (**b**) Photograph of the herniated tissue

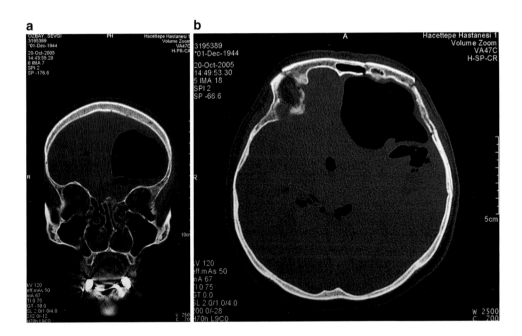

Fig. 2.11.7 (**a, b**) Air in the intracranial cavity after traumatic fracture in the anterior and posterior frontal tables and anterior skull base

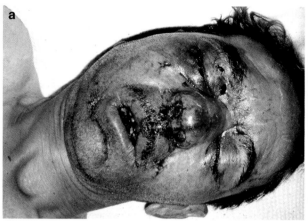

Fig. 2.11.8 (a, b) Le Fort III maxillary fracture. Extensive facial fractures may require urgent intervention to prevent respiratory obstruction. Maxillary fractures were first classified by Dr. Le Fort and this classification system was called the "Le Fort classification." In the Le Fort classification system there are three types of fractures: Le Fort I: The fracture line passes along the pyriform aperture and inferior wall of the antrum. It is a low maxillary fracture that separates the maxilla at the level of the nasal floor. Le Fort II (pyramidal fracture): The fracture line passes across the nasal bone, the frontal processes of the maxilla, and the zygomatic-maxillary junction. It separates the *central (middle)* third of face from the base of the skull. Le Fort III (craniofacial dysjunction): The facial bones separate completely from the skull base. The fracture line extends along the nasofrontal, maxillofrontal, and zygomaticofrontal sutures. These fractures are reduced with miniplates

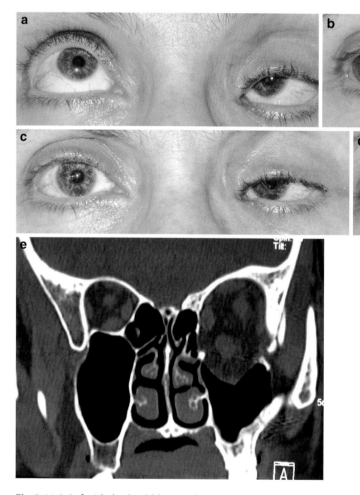

Fig. 2.11.9 Left-sided orbital blowout fracture. The soft tissue contents of the orbit have extruded into the maxillary antrum. Orbital blowout fracture is usually caused by blunt trauma to the eye globe. Increased pressure in the orbit causes fracture in the weakest part of the orbital cavity. The orbital contents extrude into the maxillary antrum. Entrapment of the inferior rectus muscle causes limitation of eye movement. Orbital herniation leads to enophthalmos on long-term follow-up. **(a–g)** After a severe maxillofacial trauma, mistreated blowout fracture resulted in enophthalmos and restriction in the mobility of the left eye. The patient recovered from diplopia after surgery (courtesy of Dr. Şener)

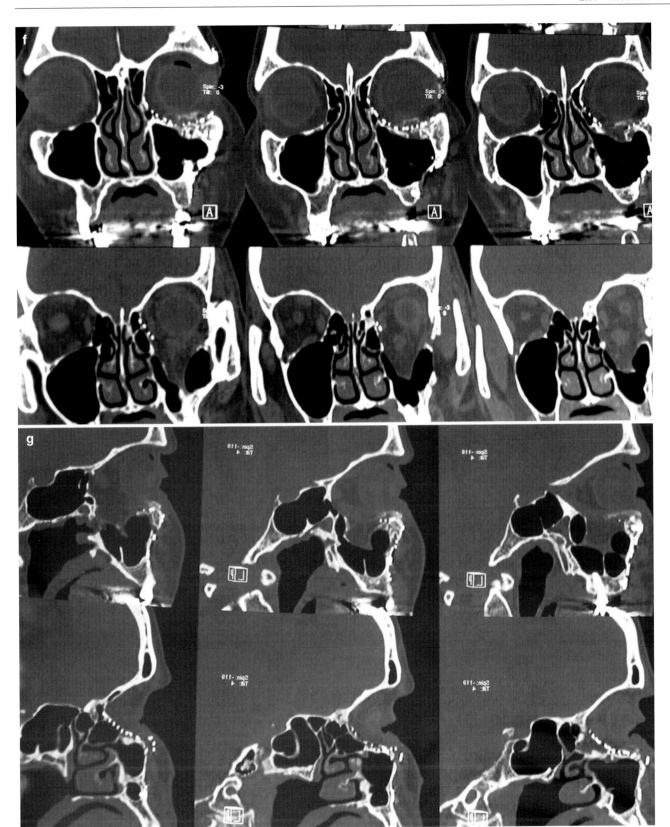

Fig. 2.11.9 (Continued)

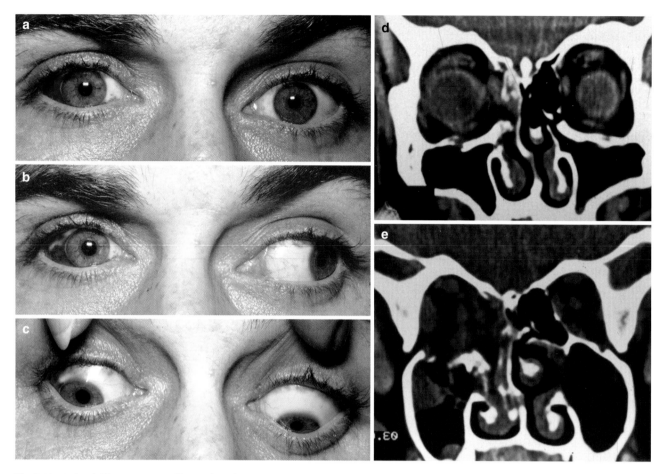

Fig. 2.11.10 (a–e) After a severe traffic accident, fracture in the medial and inferior orbital walls resulted in enophthalmos and restriction in the mobility of the right eye. Gaze to the medial and inferior sides is limited. Note the herniation of the globe to the ethmoids (courtesy of Dr. Şener)

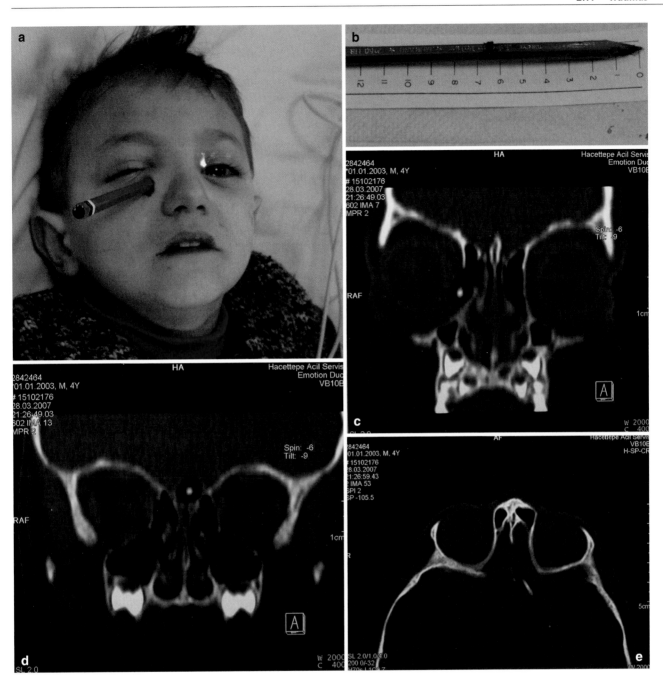

Fig. 2.11.11 Penetrating trauma to the right orbit and the intracranial cavity. The pencil was taken out, all foreign material cleaned, and CSF fistula repaired. (**a, b**) Pencil penetrating the skin just inferior and medial to the orbit. (**c–e**) Coronal and axial CT scans showing trauma to the eye and the intracranial cavity (courtesy of Tesav)

289 **2.12**

290 **Nasolacrimal obstructions**

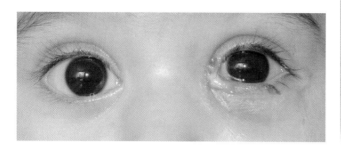

Fig. 2.12.1 Acute dacryocystitis on the left side

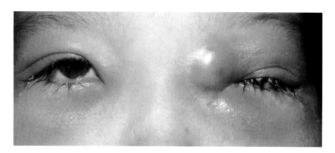

Fig. 2.12.2 Acute dacryocystitis with severe infection around the eye. Note the fluctuating mass in the left internal canthal area with hyperemia and edema around the left eye

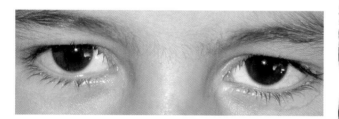

Fig. 2.12.3 Congenital dacryostenosis with lengthened fluorescein drainage time on the right side

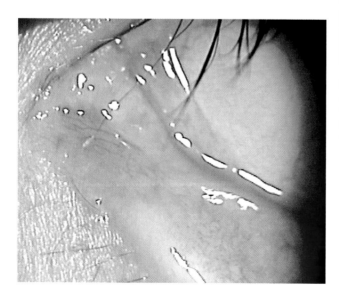

Fig. 2.12.4 Punctum agenesis on the left side

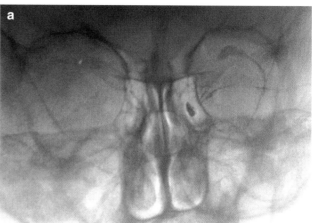

a

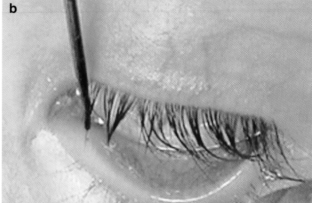

b

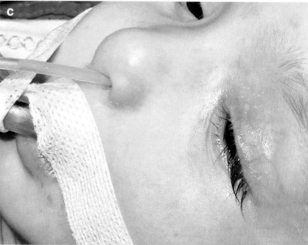

c

Fig. 2.12.5 Congenital dacryostenosis on the left side. **(a)** Macro-dacryocystography. Opaque material on the left side was not drained to the nose. Opaque material on the right side has already been drained. **(b)** Probing of the left nasolacrimal canal. **(c)** Fluorescein suctioned from the inferior meatus after injection to the nasolacrimal canal

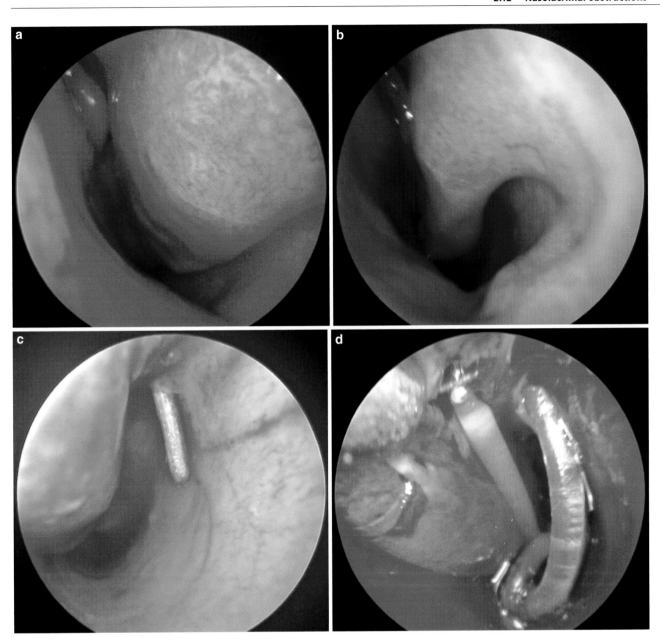

Fig. 2.12.6 Endoscopic intubation of a patient with congenital dacryostenosis on the left side. (a) Inferior turbinate. (b) Medialization of the inferior turbinate. (c) The tip of the probe in the inferior meatus.

(d) Silicon tubes tied in the inferior meatus after they have been passed through the nasolacrimal canal under endoscopic control

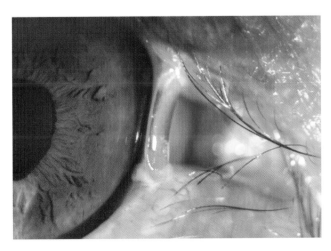

Fig. 2.12.7 The loop of the silicon tube should not be very tight in order to avoid trauma to the canaliculi

2.13

Tumors

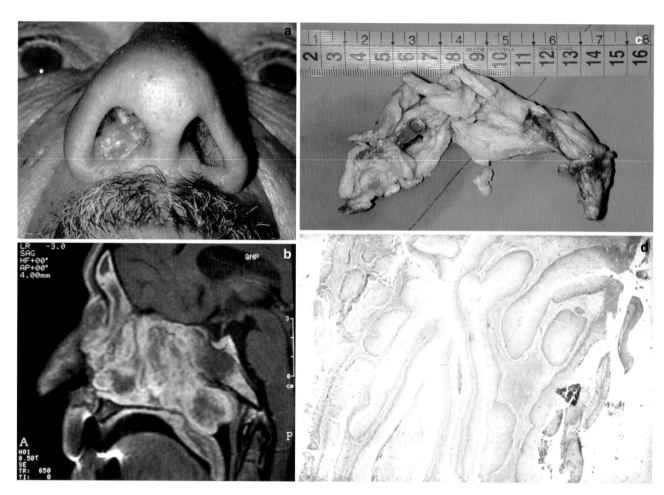

Fig. 2.13.1 Inverted papillomas generally arise from the lateral nasal wall. They are unilateral masses. In 15% of cases there may be malignant transformation. The tumor should be excised completely and sent for histological examination to check for malignant transforma- tion. Endoscopic removal is the treatment of choice. (**a**) Right-sided mass. (**b**) On sagittal MR image, the mass completely fills the nasal cavity. (**c**) Removal of the mass. (**d**) Histological picture of the inverted papilloma. Epithelium shows invaginations into the tissue

Fig. 2.13.2 Inverted papilloma that fills the nostril and is clearly visible

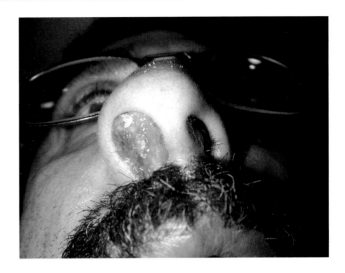

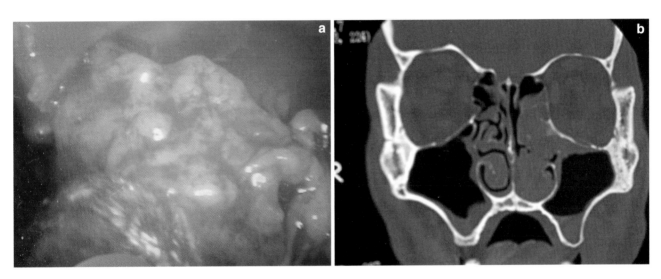

Fig. 2.13.3 Left-sided inverted papilloma. (**a**) Endoscopic appearance. (**b**) Coronal CT shows extension to the upper wall of the maxillary antrum

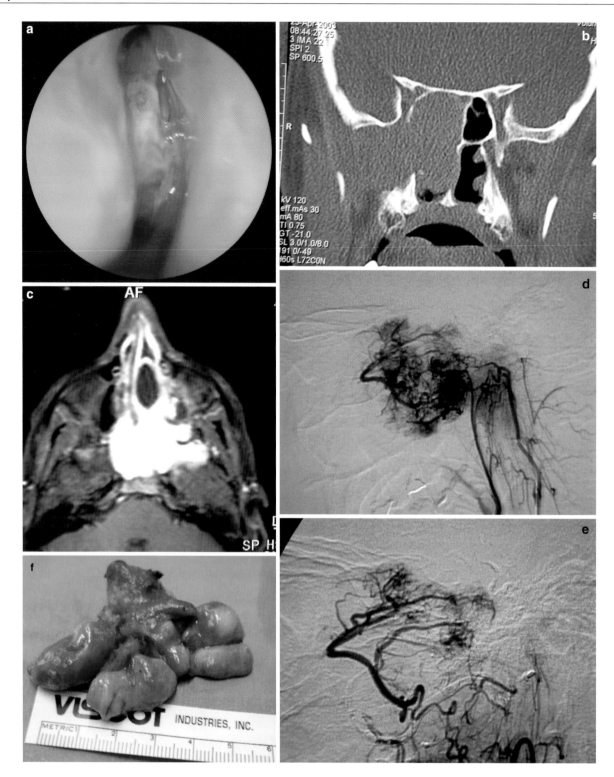

Fig. 2.13.4 Juvenile nasopharyngeal angiofibroma. It usually arises superior and posterior to the sphenopalatine foramen. It only occurs in male adolescents. These patients present with the complaint of nasal obstruction and bleeding. (**a**) Endoscopic view. (**b**) On coronal CT scan. widening of pterygomaxillary fissure is diagnostic. (**c**) Axial CT shows extension to the infratemporal fossa. (**d**) Angiography shows the hypervascularity of the tumor. (**e**) Embolization helps the surgeon to operate in a less bloody field. No vascularity after embolization is seen. (**f**) Endoscopic surgery is the treatment of choice. Specimen after total removal of the tumor

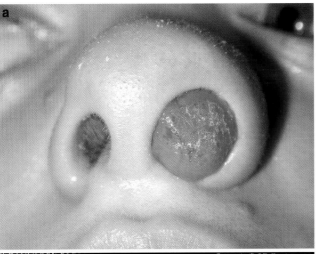

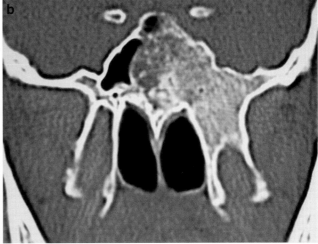

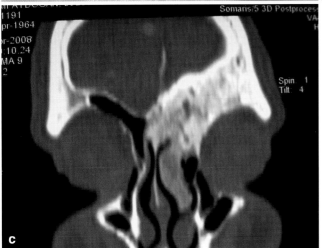

Fig. 2.13.5 Fibrous dysplasia is a fibro-osseous disease of the facial skeleton. It usually appears during the first two decades of life. On CT scan, ground glass presentation due to a mixture of fibrous and osseous components is characteristic of this tumor. If it does not cause any deformity or functional disorder, no surgery is required. **(a)** Fibrous dysplasia filling the left nostril completely. **(b)** Coronal CT showing fibrous dysplasia in the sphenoid bone. **(c)** Coronal CT showing fibrous dysplasia in the frontal bone

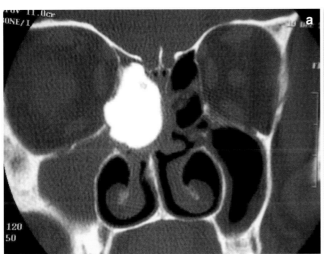

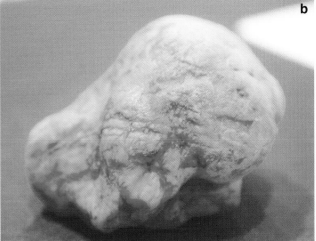

Fig. 2.13.6 Osteomas are common benign tumors of the sinuses. They occur most frequently in the frontoethmoid region. **(a)** Coronal CT showing osteoma in the right ethmoid area. **(b)** The specimen after removal

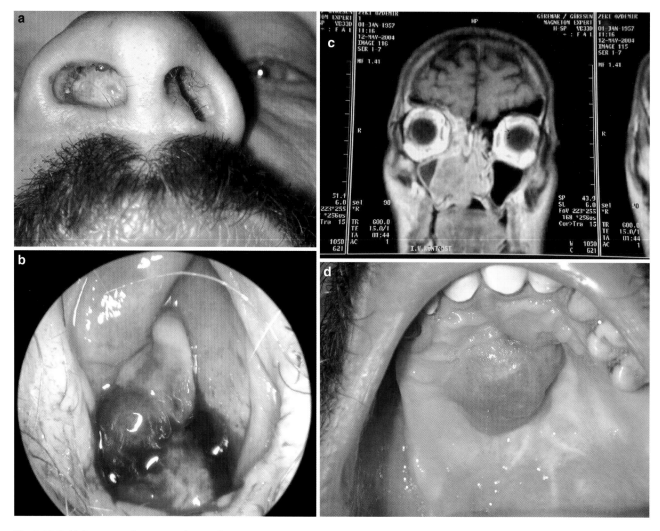

Fig. 2.13.7 Malignant melanoma in the nasal cavity. **(a)** Mass in the right nasal cavity. **(b)** Pigmented mass after cleaning of purulent material. **(c)** Coronal MR image shows mass filling the ethmoids and maxillary sinus and extending to the palate. **(d)** Mass in the hard palate. Mass in the nasal cavity has eroded the palatal bone

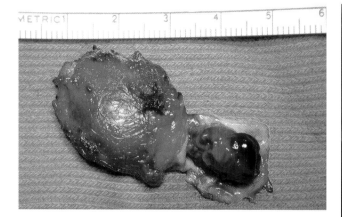

Fig. 2.13.8 Specimen of mucosal malignant melanoma in the nose after excision with safe margins. Malignant melanoma of the sinonasal tract comprises 1–2% of all melanomas. A pigmented polyp may be a malignant melanoma

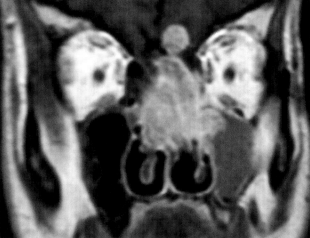

Fig. 2.13.9 A unilateral mass in the nose that bleeds spontaneously should arouse the suspicion of malignancy. Esthesioneuroblastoma is an uncommon tumor that arises in the olfactory epithelium. These tumors very often invade the cranium. To show the intracranial extension, MR imaging is necessary

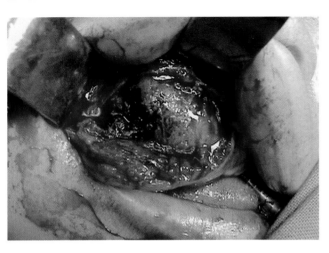

Fig. 2.13.10 Neuroblastomas are sarcomas of nervous system origin affecting mostly infants and children up to 10 years of age

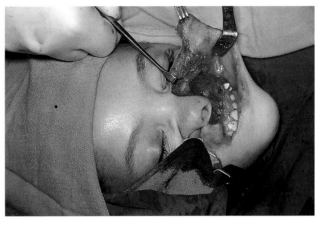

Fig. 2.13.12 Lateral rhinotomy approach had been used for removal of tumors of the nasal cavity and paranasal sinuses. In the lateral rhinotomy approach, an incision is made along the nasofacial sulcus. This incision is extended into the nasal cavity along the nasolabial sulcus. The nasal flap is prepared and rotated upward and medially. Due to poor cosmetic results, this technique was replaced by other techniques

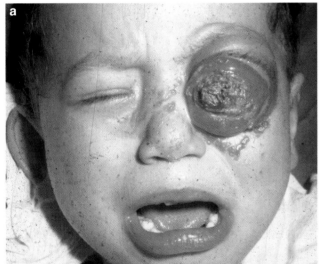

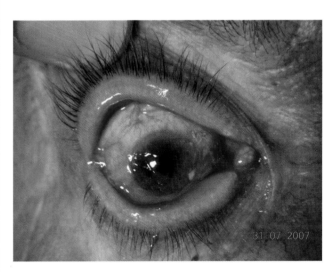

Fig. 2.13.13 Epidermoid carcinoma in the medial canthus of the right eye (courtesy of Dr. Kıratlı)

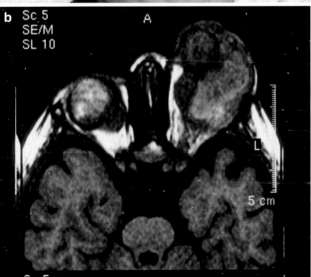

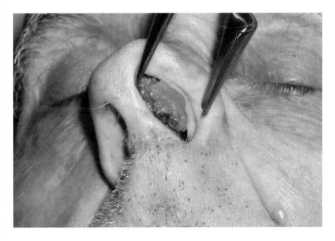

Fig. 2.13.11 (a) Retinoblastoma is the most frequent intraocular malignant tumor in childhood affecting mostly infants and children up to 3 years of age. (b) Axial MR image (courtesy of Dr. Kıratlı)

Fig. 2.13.14 Epidermoid carcinoma in the left nasal vestibule

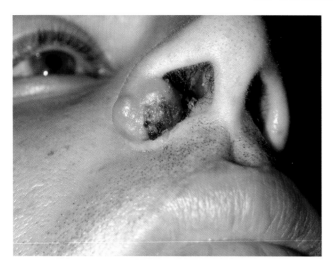

Fig. 2.13.15 Epidermoid carcinoma in the right nasal ala

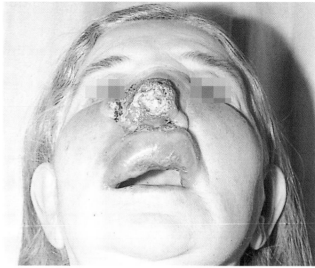

Fig. 2.13.17 Epidermoid carcinoma that invades the nasal tip and nasal cavities

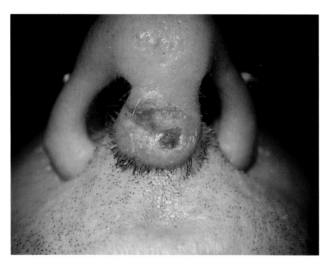

Fig. 2.13.16 Epidermoid carcinoma invading the columella and extending into both nasal cavities

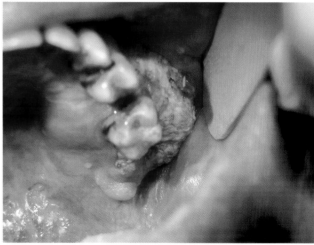

Fig. 2.13.18 Epidermoid carcinoma filling the left gingivobuccal sulcus and invading the left maxillary sinus

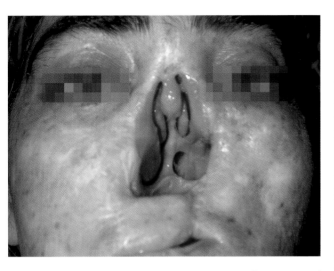

Fig. 2.13.19 Total nose excision due to squamous cell carcinoma of the nose

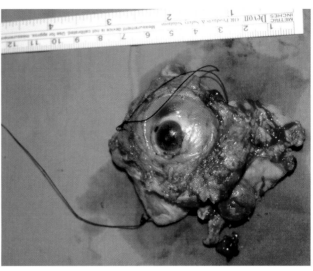

Fig. 2.13.21 Excision of the tumor with exenteration of the eye

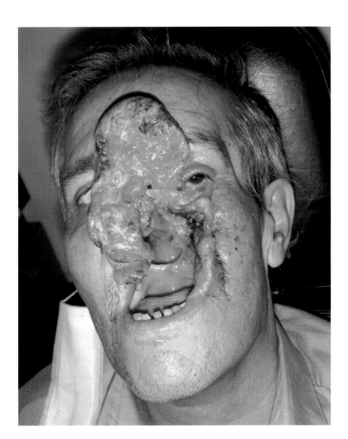

Fig. 2.13.20 Epidermoid carcinoma causing destruction of the face

THROAT & NECK

CONTENTS

T. Metln Önerci: *Diagnosis in Otorhinolaryngology*
DOI: 10.1007/978-3-642-00499-5_3, © Springer-Verlag Berlin Heidelberg 2009

3.1

Acute Tonsillopharyngitis

The term sore throat is used to define all kinds of acute inflammatory symptoms in the throat. Sore throat is more common in children than in adults. Children may experience six to eight upper respiratory tract infections. Half of these infections are associated with pharyngitis. A viral pharyngitis is frequently accompanied by a runny nose and cough.

Table 3.1.1 Etiology of sore throats

Acute pharyngitis
Acute tonsillitis
Lingual tonsillitis
Peritonsillar abscess
Vincent's angina
Diphtheria
Candidiasis
Infectious mononucleosis
Acute leukaemia

In normal children both viral (15–40%) and bacterial infections (30–40%) are common.In adults infections are generally viral. Group A beta-hemolytic streptococcus (GABHS) is generally the primary causative organism rather than a secondary invader. GABHS infections are rarely seen in adults and in children younger than 2 years.

It is important to differentiate GABHS infections in children. The antibiotic therapy should be started within 9 days after the onset of infection to prevent potential cardiac and renal complications. It is not possible to make a diagnosis of GABHS infection by clinical examination alone. Throat swabs are necessary to identify *Streptococcus* (Fig. 3.1.1). Generally, a cherry red tongue and perioral pallor suggest GABHS infection. In infectious mononucleosis, the cervical lymph nodes are enlarged and petechial hemorrhages may be seen on the palate. In some patients, hepatosplenomegaly may be palpable. A positive Paul-Bunnell test result or identification of atypical lymphocytes in the peripheral blood is diagnostic for infectious mononucleosis. Administration of ampicillin in infectious mononucleosis cases causes skin rash. Biopsy of lymph nodes during acute infectious mononucleosis may lead to an erroneous diagnosis of lymphoma. In GABHS infections the primary antibiotic treatment is penicillin. Antibiotic treatment should be continued at least for 10 days. To date, there is no vaccine developed against GABHS.

In immunocompromised patients fungal infections such as candidiasis should be kept in mind.

The first signs of acute leukemia may be oral lesions. Enlarged tonsils with ulcerative lesions, petechial lesions and bleeding in the oral cavity, gingival ulcerations, a low-grade fever, and cervical lymphadenopathy should alert the physician to the possibility of acute leukemia.

Is penicillin prophylaxis necessary in recurrent GABHS infections?

Unless there is an anamnesis of previous acute rheumatic fever, there is no evidence that penicillin prophylaxis prevents recurrent attacks of acute tonsillopharyngitis.

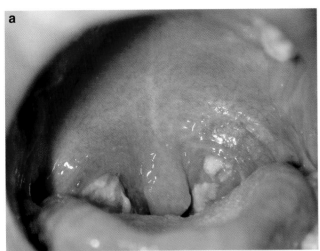

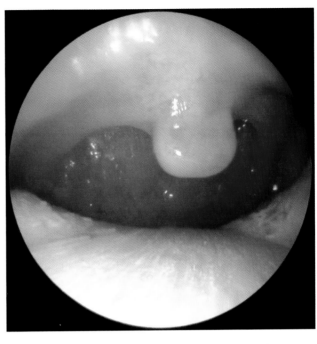

Fig. 3.1.2 Acute pharyngitis. The pharyngeal mucosa is hyperemic and edematous. The patient shows all the symptoms and signs of infection and sore throat

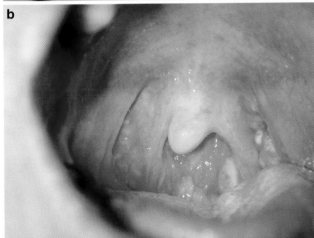

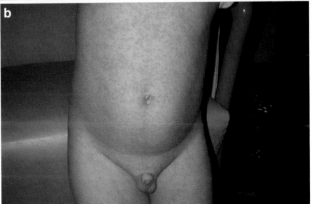

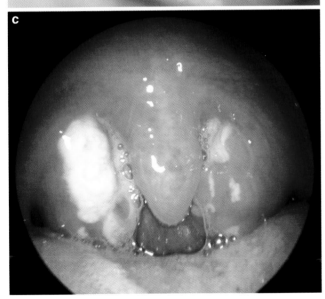

Fig. 3.1.1 (**a**) Acute tonsillitis due to group A beta-hemolytic strep-tococcal (GABHS) infection. (**b**) Acute tonsillitis and pharyngitis. Exu-dative lesions are seen both on the tonsils and pharyngeal mucosa. (**c**) Acute tonsillitis in a patient with infectious mononucleosis

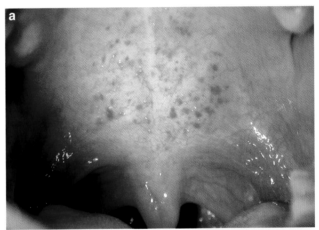

Fig. 3.1.3 (**a**) Petechial hemorrhages are seen on the soft palate in a patient with infectious mononucleosis. (**b**) Ampicillin rash. Ampicil-lin treatment in patients with infectious mononucleosis causes rash. The ampicillin rash resembles measles

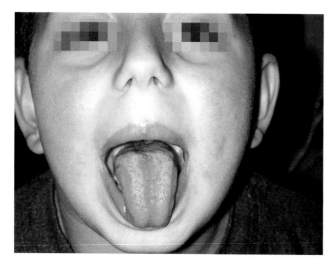

Fig. 3.1.4 Generally a cherry red tongue and perioral pallor suggest GABHS infection

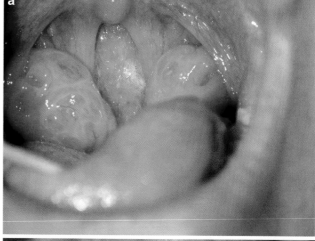

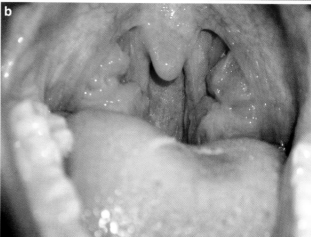

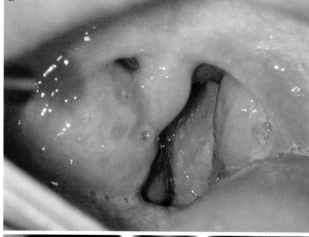

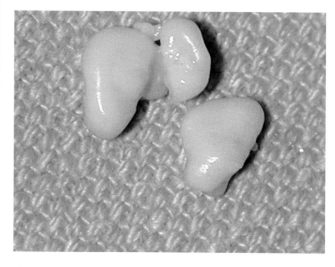

Fig. 3.1.6 (a, b) Chronic tonsillitis. There is no straightforward diagnosis for chronic tonsillitis. Deep tonsillar crypts, white debris in these crypts, and the vascularization of the anterior pillars are seen. This white debris consisting of stagnated food remnants in the crypts may cause halitosis

Fig. 3.1.5 Hypertrophic tonsils. **(a)** The right tonsil is more hypertrophic than the left one. **(b)** Kissing tonsils. The tonsils cause obstruction and sleep apnea

Fig. 3.1.7 Tonsilloliths. Stagnated food remnants may stay in the crypts for a long period, become hardened, and look like small stones called tonsilloliths

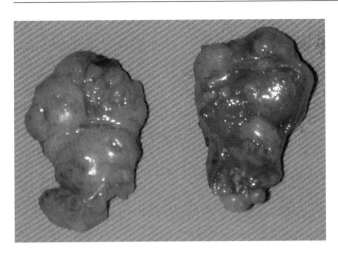

Fig. 3.1.8 Tonsils removed with their capsules after tonsillectomy

Table 3.1.3 Contraindications to tonsillectomy

Bleeding disorders
Recent acute infection
Children under the age of 3 years
Young children weighing less than 15 kg have a greater risk associated with blood loss

Table 3.1.2 Indications of tonsillectomy

Recurrent acute tonsillitis (more than five episodes in 1 year, five attacks per year for two consecutive years, or three attacks per year for three consecutive years)
Recurrent acute tonsillitis with recurrent febrile seizures or cardiac complications
Chronic tonsillitis
Peritonsillar abscess
Obstructive tonsillar hypertrophy causing disturbances with respiration and nutrition
Obstructive sleep apnea syndrome
Asymmetric growth or tonsillar lesion suggestive of neoplasm

3.2

Adenoids

Adenoids are an accumulation of lymphoid tissue located at the posterosuperior wall of the nasopharynx above the level of soft palate. Recurrent upper respiratory tract infections cause adenoids to enlarge. Adenoids reach their greatest size at the age of 6 years and then gradually regress. If adenoids obstruct the eustachian tube they may cause otitis media with effusion. Adenoids also serve as a reservoir for microorganisms and may be the cause of recurrent infections. Adenoids may cause nasal obstruction and sleep apnea. Adenoid hypertrophy alone or together with tonsillar hypertrophy with chronic mouth breathing may cause craniofacial growth abnormalities. The anterior facial height is increased, the midface is flat, and the palate is highly arched. This typical facial appearance is called adenoid face. If adenoid face develops it is difficult to correct this skeletal deformity. Adenoidectomy will not reverse dental changes that have already occurred. Orthodontic assistance is important but it is not always helpful. Maxillofacial surgery may be needed for correction in some cases.

In adults, nasopharyngeal carcinoma should be suspected if nasal obstruction is associated with a unilateral serous otitis media.

Fiberoptic or rigid endoscopes provide sufficient visualization of the nasopharynx. Lateral X-rays may show the size of the adenoids and the degree of obstruction. Correct positioning of the child is very important. A wrongly angled X-ray may erroneously point to large adenoids. Plain X-rays should be avoided in children due to the harmful effects of radiation. Endoscopy may help rule out other diseases such as Thornwald cysts or malignancy causing nasal obstruction.

Adenoidectomy should be undertaken in patients with symptoms. Submucous cleft palate should always be checked for before the operation and adenoidectomy should be avoided in the presence of a submucous cleft. A bifid uvula may be a sign of a possible submucous palatal cleft. The adenoids are curetted. Since surgery is blind and the adenoid tissue does not have a capsule as in the tonsils, complete removal of the adenoids is almost impossible.

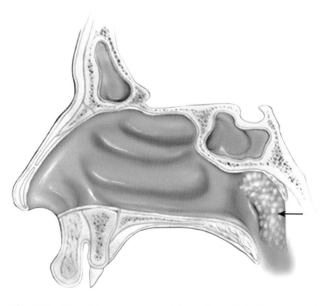

Fig. 3.2.1 Adenoids are an accumulation of lymphoid tissue located at the posterosuperior wall of the nasopharynx above the level of the soft palate

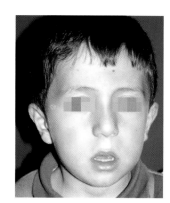

Fig. 3.2.3 Adenoid face is a typical facial appearance with increased anterior facial height and flat midface

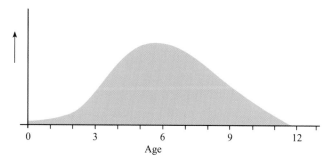

Fig. 3.2.2 Adenoids reach their greatest size at the age of 6 years and then gradually regress

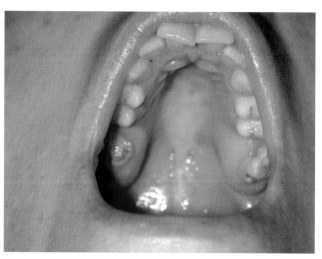

Fig. 3.2.4 The palate is high arched in children with adenoidal hypertrophy

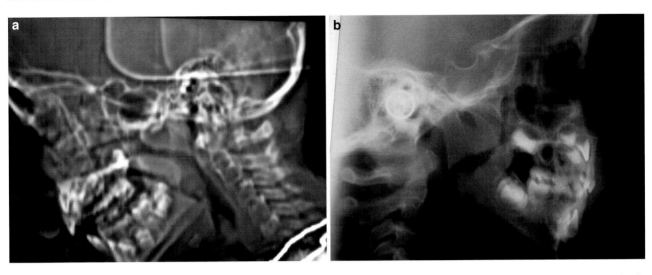

Fig. 3.2.5 Lateral X-ray of the postnasal space. **(a)** Adenoid tissue is not obstructing the airway; **(b)** adenoid tissue is almost completely obstructing the airway

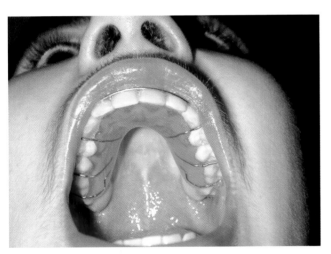

Fig. 3.2.6 Orthodontic apparatus to correct hard palate deformity due to adenoid hypertrophy

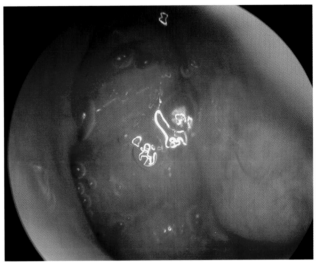

Fig. 3.2.8 Endoscopic photograph of adenoidal hypertrophy

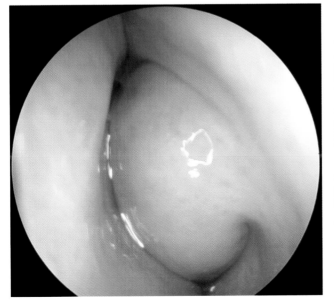

Fig. 3.2.7 Inferior turbinate hypertrophies may accompany adenoid hypertrophy. Sometimes they are the only cause of nasal obstruction

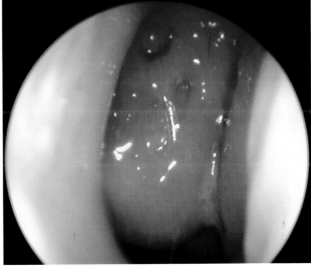

Fig. 3.2.9 Endoscopic photograph of Thornwald cyst

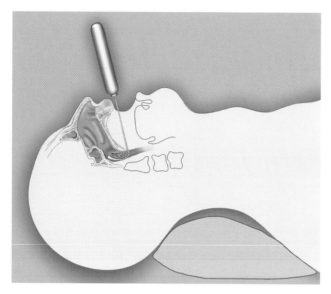

Fig. 3.2.10 Adenoidectomy technique

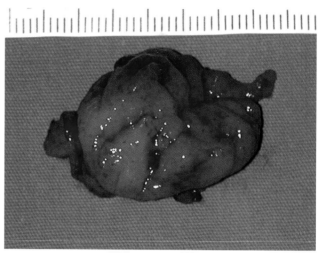

Fig. 3.2.11 Adenoid tissue after removal

Table 3.2.1 Indications for adenoidectomy

Adenoid hypertrophy with chronic mouth breathing
Adenoid hypertrophy with sleep apnea
Chronic adenoiditis with middle ear effusions
Suspicion of a nasopharyngeal malignancy (for biopsy purposes)

Table 3.2.2 Contraindications for adenoidectomy

Bleeding disorders
Recent upper respiratory tract infection
Submucosal cleft palate

3.3

Snoring

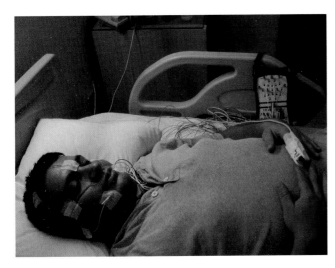

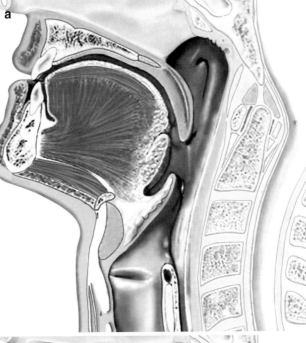

Fig. 3.3.1 Snoring is the sound created by vibrations of the pharyngeal structures. Apnea is the cessation of breathing for more than 10 s. Sleep apnea is defined as more than five episodes of apnea per hour. Apnea may be central or obstructive. Central apnea is caused by a lack of drive in the central nervous system (CNS). The majority of apneas are obstructive. Some patients may have a mixed type of apnea. Since severe apnea may have serious cardiac and CNS complications, sleep apnea is a disease to be treated. The gold standard in the diagnosis of sleep apnea is polysomnography

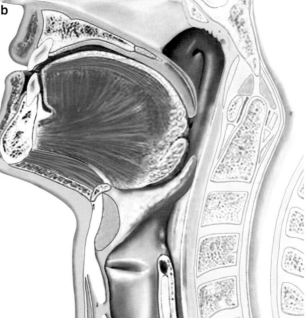

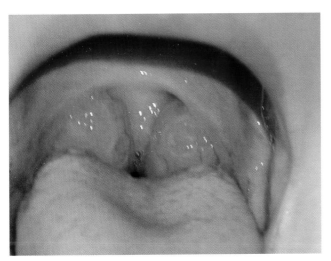

Fig. 3.3.3 (a) Tongue base is at its normal position. (b) Tongue base can be displaced posteriorly, narrowing the oropharynx and causing snoring and apnea

Fig. 3.3.2 Hypertrophic tonsils may be the only cause of snoring and apnea. Tonsillectomy may solve the problem

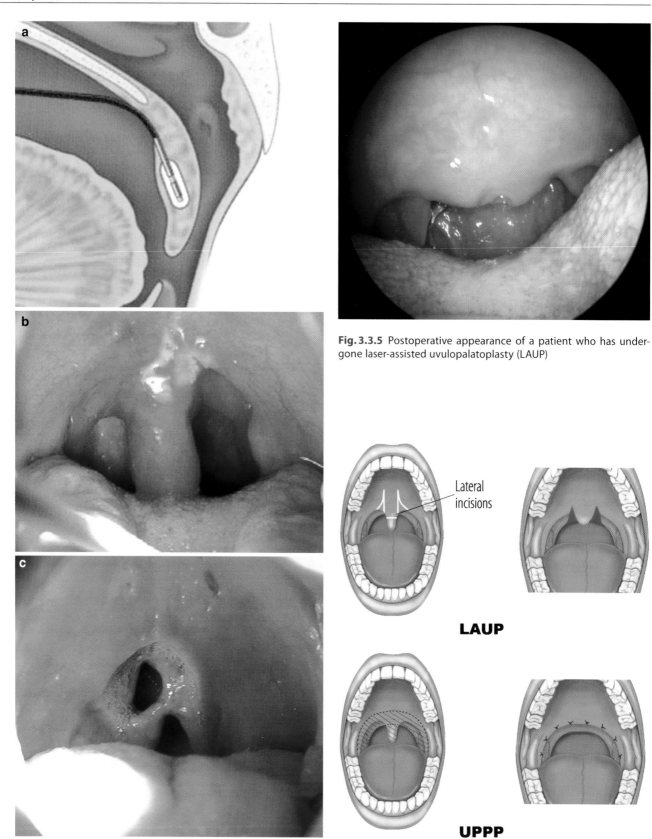

Fig. 3.3.5 Postoperative appearance of a patient who has undergone laser-assisted uvulopalatoplasty (LAUP)

Lateral incisions

LAUP

UPPP

Excised area in UPPP

Fig. 3.3.4 Radiosurgery of the palate. **(a)** Radiosurgery produces fibrosis in the soft palate and increases the stiffness of the soft palate. **(b)** Applications at the base of the uvula may cause edema of the uvula. **(c)** If too much energy is delivered at the same point it may cause perforation of the soft palate

Fig. 3.3.6 Schematic view of laser-assisted uvulopalatoplasty and classic uvulopalatopharyngoplasty (*UPPP*) with tonsillectomy

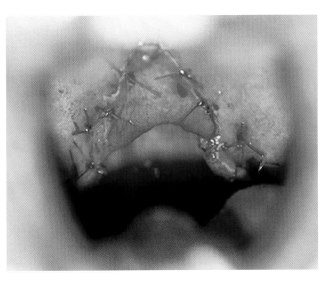

Fig. 3.3.7 Uvulopalatal flap (courtesy of Çelikoyar). After the mucosa of the lingual surface of the uvula and some of the soft palate are stripped away, the uvula is reflected back toward the soft palate and fixed into its new position

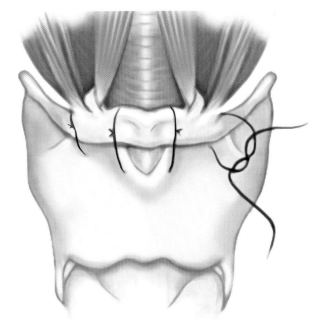

Fig. 3.3.9 Hyoid suspension operation. The hyoid bone is fixated on the upper edge of the thyroid cartilage with a steel wire suture. This brings the tongue base anteriorly and caudally. The hyoid suspension operation is believed to prevent the hypopharyngeal collapse of the tongue muscles

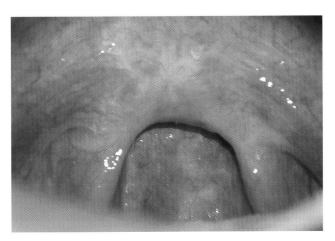

Fig. 3.3.8 Appearance of soft palate after classic UPPP

Table 3.3.1 The questions to be asked in a patient with obstructive sleep apnea syndrome

Do you snore?
Does your family complain about your snoring?
Does your spouse say that your breathing stops at certain intervals?
Do you wake up during your sleep with air hunger?
Do you have morning headaches?
Do you feel tired in the morning when you wake up?
Do you have daytime somnolence?
Do you feel sleepy at work?
Do you fall asleep while watching TV?
Do you fall asleep while sitting?

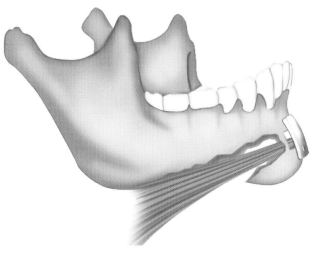

Fig. 3.3.10 Genioglossus advancement technique. By advancing the genial tubercle and genioglossus muscle, the hypopharyngeal airway is enlarged and the collapse is prevented

3.4

Temporomandibular Joint

Temporomandibular joint (TMJ) problems are very common in the population. Patients may present with the symptoms of pain, joint noises, locking, and limited opening. Pain may be due to either the joint problem itself or the related muscles of mastication. Pain localized in front of the tragus is probably TMJ pain. Pain localized to the mandibular or temple area may be myofascial pain. Myofascial pain is more severe in the mornings because of the activities of the muscle during the night, such as clenching or grinding the teeth. Clicking is related to the anterior dislocation of the disc. Only clicking does not require any treatment.

The primary management of TMJ disorders is reassurance of the patient that there is no serious underlying condition. Muscle relaxants, nonsteroidal anti-inflammatory drugs, and heat application may improve the symptoms. The patient should be evaluated by a dentist regarding the occlusion, and occlusal or anterior repositioning splints may be advised to be worn at night.

a

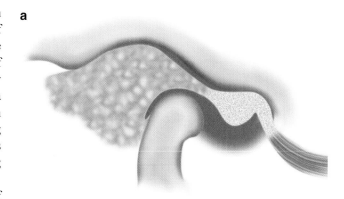

b

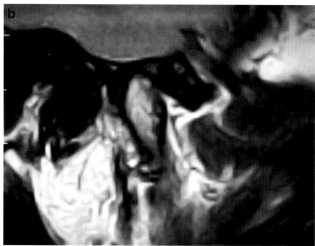

Fig. 3.4.3 (a) Schematic representation of TMJ anterior disc dislocation with reduction. The disc is normally placed between the condyle and the articular fossa. **(b)** MR examination; sagittal view of the TMJ. The disk is located anterior to the articular fossa

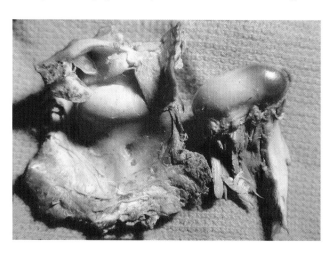

Fig. 3.4.1 Cadaver dissection. Temporomandibular joint (TMJ) disc and condyle with attached superior pterygoid muscle. The disc of the TMJ is continuous with the superior pterygoid muscle fibers. Some of the fibers of the pterygoid muscle attach to the condyle as well. This allows the joint to work in a synchronous way

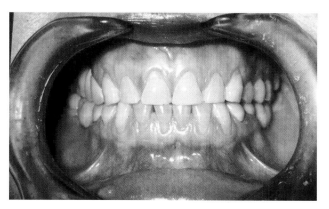

Fig. 3.4.2 Normal occlusion is necessary for normal TMJ function

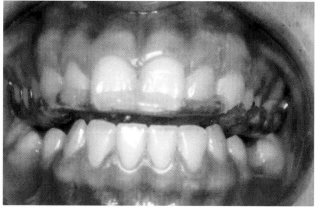

Fig. 3.4.4 Occlusal splints help to keep the jaws in normal occlusion

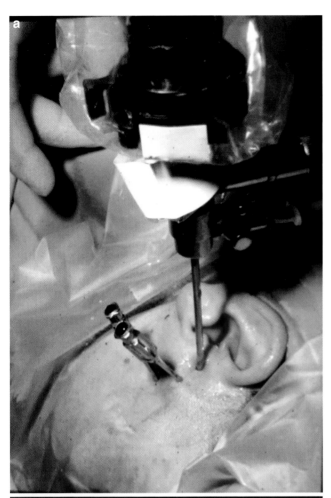

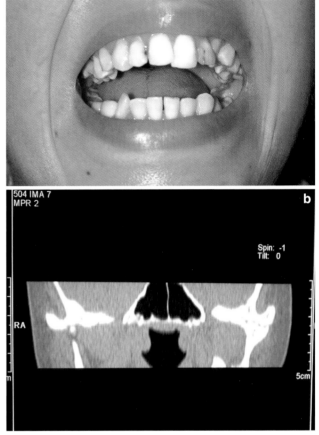

Fig. 3.4.6 (a) In TMJ ankylosis, opening of the mouth is limited. (b) On coronal CT, left-sided ankylosis of the TMJ is seen

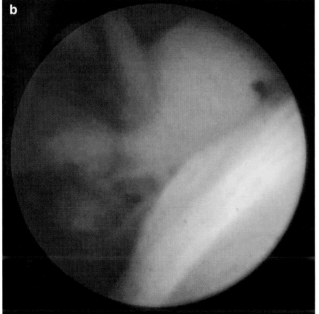

Fig. 3.4.5 (a) Surgical arthroscopy. (b) Appearance of the inside of the TMJ and avascular disc in white color

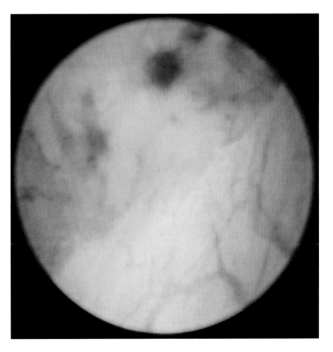

Fig. 3.4.7 Arthroscopic view of TMJ anterior disc dislocation. Avascular white disc has escaped to the anterior recess and the posterior ligament lies between the condyle and the articular fossa

3.5

Airway Obstructions

Table 3.5.1 Differential diagnosis in acute epiglottitis and acute laryngotracheobronchitis

	Acute epiglottitis	Acute laryngotracheobronchitis
Pathogen	*Haemophilus influenzae* type B	Viruses
Age group	2–6	1–3
Incidence	10%	90%
Onset	Rapid (hours)	Slow (days)
General condition	Severe systemic toxicity	Satisfactory
Cough	Absent	Barking cough
Dysphagia	Severe	Absent
Drooling	Marked	Absent
Stridor	Inspiratory	Biphasic
Fever	>39°C	<39°C
Posture	Sitting up	Lying back
Voice	Muffled (not hoarse)	Hoarse
X-ray	Thumbprint sign	Steeple sign

Croup is infection of the larynx resulting in airway obstruction and stridor. Stridor is the high-frequency sound created during inspiration and expiration. Narrowing of the trachea or the larynx produces inspiratory stridor. Bronchial narrowing produces expiratory stridor. Stridor is not a disease or a diagnosis but only a symptom. Under the term croup, acute epiglottitis, acute laryngotracheobronchitis, and bacterial tracheitis can be mentioned. Acute laryngotracheobronchitis is the most common infection causing airway obstruction in children. Acute epiglottitis has a very rapid onset and is highly lethal if not diagnosed and treated immediately. Introduction of the HIB vaccine has reduced the incidence of acute epiglottitis by more than 90%. Clinical features of the differential diagnosis between acute epiglottitis and acute laryngotracheobronchitis can be seen in Table 3.5.1.

Bacterial tracheitis is generally seen from infancy to adulthood. The most commonly isolated pathogen is *Staphylococcus aureus*. The initial clinical course is similar to that seen in croup. The tracheal mucosa is edematous and diffusely ulcerated causing tracheal narrowing. Thick purulent secretions partially obstruct the tracheal lumen. Thick purulent secretions in the trachea sometimes cause severe airway obstruction. When needed, endotracheal intubation and repeated suction of the secretions should be performed.

Spasmodic croup must be differentiated from croup. It is seen between the ages of 1–5 years. Its onset is rapid, starting usually in the evening. There is no associated infection. Humidity relieves the symptoms.

Laryngomalacia is the most common cause of stridor in infants and is the most common congenital laryngeal abnormality. The epiglottis is omega shaped. The aryepiglottic folds are tall, foreshortened, and thin and the arytenoids are large with redundant mucosa. The main theory of its cause is cartilaginous immaturity. The other theory is neuromuscular control abnormalities. The disease is generally self-limiting. However, in severe laryngomalacia surgical therapy may be necessary.

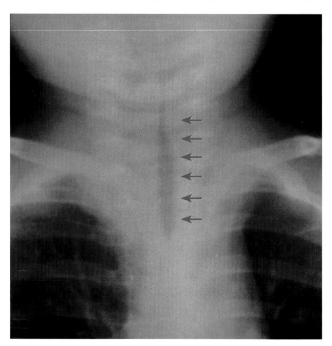

Fig. 3.5.1 Steeple sign in a child with acute laryngitis

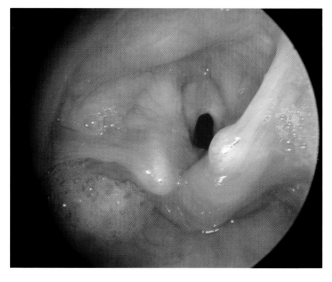

Fig. 3.5.2 Neonates with webs present with respiratory obstruction. The degree of obstruction is related to the size of the web (courtesy of Dr. Unal)

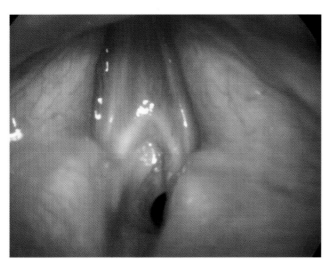

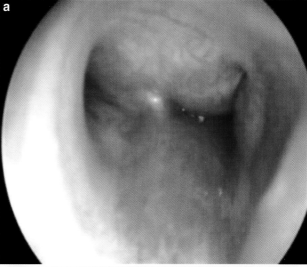

Fig. 3.5.3 Laryngeal web almost completely obstructing the airway. In severe respiratory distress, the airway must be secured either by intubation or tracheotomy. Thin webs can be opened by CO_2 laser. For thicker webs open surgery may be needed (courtesy of Dr. Unal)

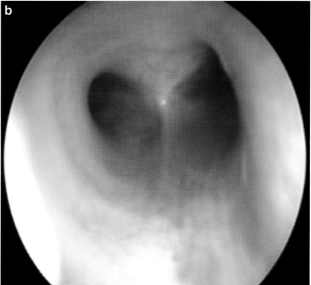

Fig. 3.5.5 **(a)** Tracheal hemangioma before and **(b)** after steroid treatment. Steroid treatment for young patients under 1 year of age may be useful (courtesy of Dr. Unal)

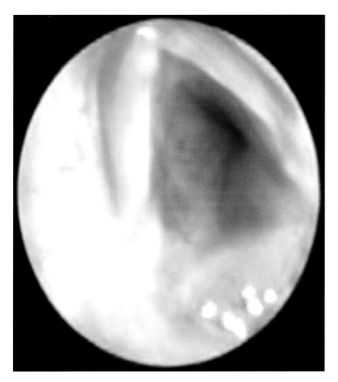

Fig. 3.5.4 Subglottic hemangiomas are the most common congenital tumors causing stridor. Subglottic and tracheal hemangiomas are generally asymptomatic at birth. Later they may become symptomatic. These tumors may regress spontaneously. In obstructing cases tracheotomy may be considered (courtesy of Dr. Unal)

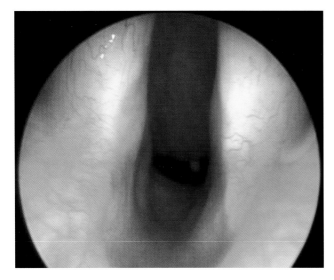

Fig.3.5.6 Congenital subglottic stenosis obstructing the airway. Subglottic stenosis may be congenital, but it is usually due to trauma of prolonged endotracheal intubation (courtesy of Dr. Unal)

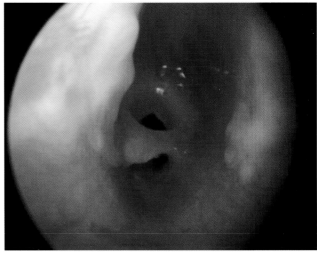

Fig.3.5.7 Early-stage subglottic stenosis due to prolonged intubation (courtesy of Dr. Unal)

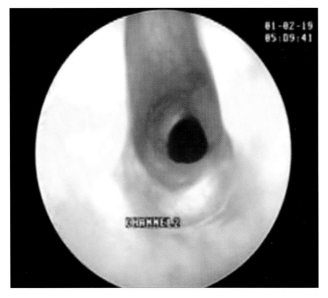

Fig.3.5.8 Subglottic stenosis due to prolonged intubation (courtesy of Dr. Unal)

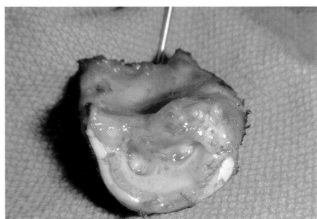

Fig.3.5.9 Tracheal resection due to subglottic stenosis (courtesy of Dr. Unal)

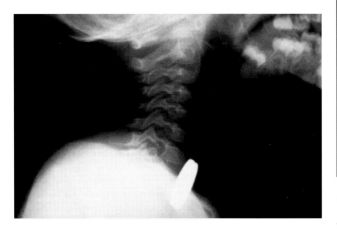

Fig.3.5.10 A foreign body (a coin) in the esophagus (courtesy of Dr. Unal)

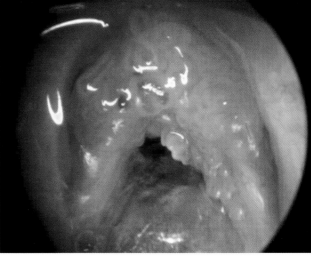

Fig.3.5.11 Juvenile laryngeal papillomatosis is the most common benign tumor of the larynx. It is caused by the human papilloma virus. CO_2 laser is of great help in the excision of papillomas. Many cases resolve by early adulthood

3.6

Hoarseness

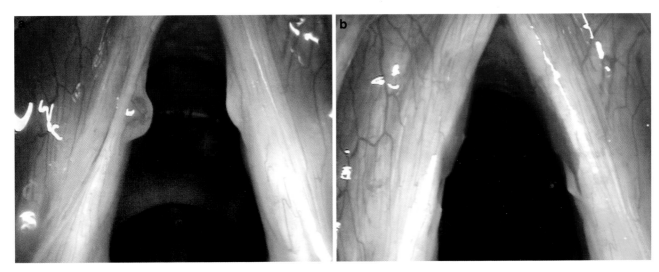

Fig. 3.6.1 **(a)** Vocal nodules are bilateral lesions at the vibratory surface of the vocal cords at the junction of the anterior one-third and posterior two-thirds. This is the area of maximum trauma at higher pitch levels during shouting and singing. Misuse of the voice is the main reason for nodules. Voice therapy is the main treatment modality. With voice therapy, 80% of vocal nodules resolve. If voice therapy fails, vocal nodules may be excised by a direct microlaryngoscopic approach. **(b)** After excision of the nodules

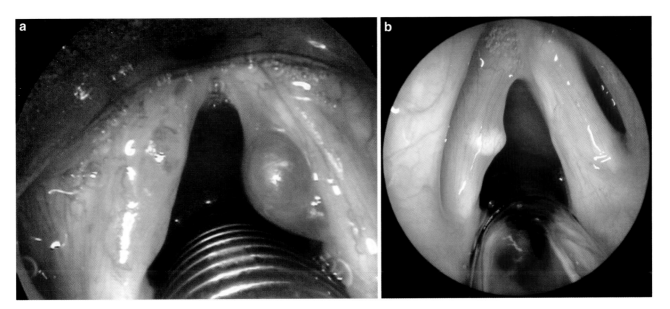

Fig. 3.6.2 **(a)** Right hemorrhagic vocal cord nodule at the junction of the anterior one-third and posterior two-thirds of the vocal cord. **(b)** Cyst at the middle of the left vocal cord. Vocal cord cysts can occur at any location on the vocal cord, and vocal abuse and gastroesophageal reflux play an important role. The cyst is evacuated through an incision without removing any mucosa

Fig. 3.6.3 Vocal polyps move in and out during respiration. **(a)** Inspiration, **(b)** expiration (courtesy of Dr. Yılmaz)

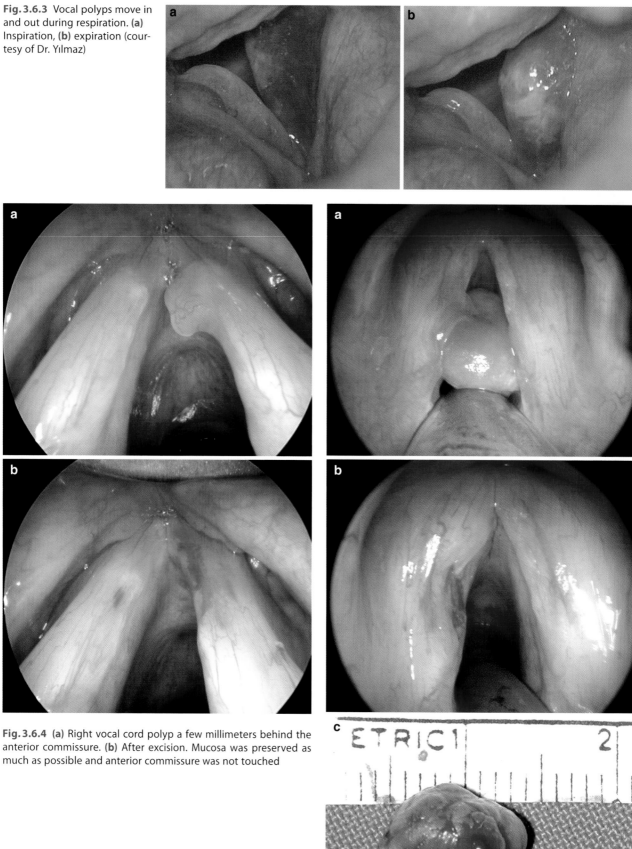

Fig. 3.6.4 (a) Right vocal cord polyp a few millimeters behind the anterior commissure. **(b)** After excision. Mucosa was preserved as much as possible and anterior commissure was not touched

Fig. 3.6.5 (a–c) Vocal cord polyps are usually single lesions which can occur anywhere on the vocal cord. The treatment is microlaryngoscopic removal of the polyps

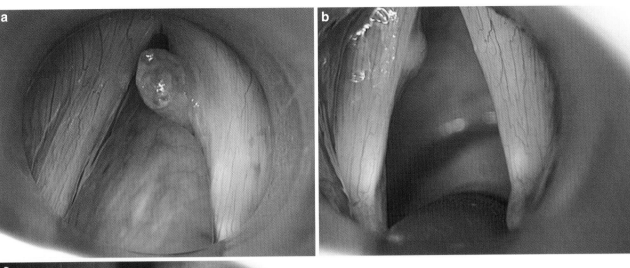

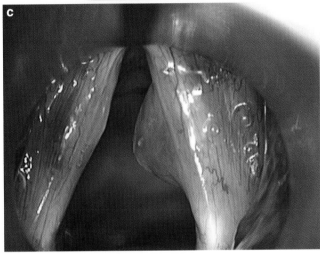

Fig. 3.6.6 (a–c) Wide base vocal cord polyps (courtesy of Dr. Yılmaz)

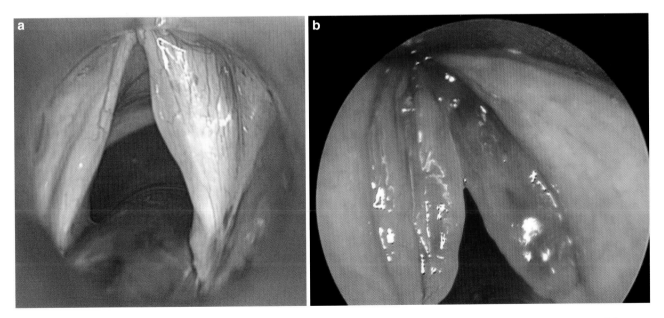

Fig. 3.6.7 (a, b) Reinke edema is the accumulation of fluid in the subepithelial space of Reinke. It is generally due to vocal abuse and smoking. If voice therapy fails, the fluid in the subepithelial space is drained through an incision without removing any overlying mucosa (courtesy of Dr. Yılmaz)

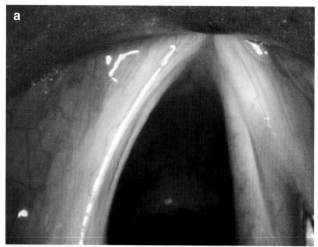

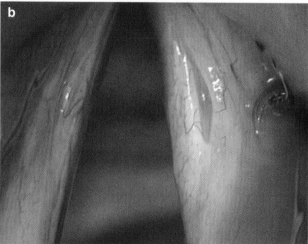

Fig. 3.6.8 (a, b) Sulcus vocalis is a longitudinal groove on the vocal cord epithelium inward toward the vocal ligament

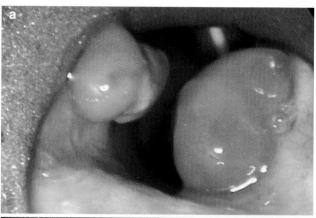

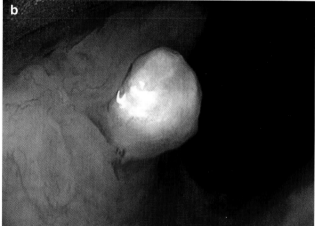

Fig. 3.6.10 Vocal cord granulomas may be unilateral or bilateral. Gastroesophageal reflux, vocal abuse, and intubation trauma are the main causative factors. Anesthetic tubes may cause trauma to the mucosa overlying the vocal process of the arytenoid cartilage. Prolonged vocal abuse may cause ulceration of the epithelium over the vocal process (contact ulcers). Treatment involves management of gastroesophageal reflux, elimination of vocal abuse, and microlaryngeal excision of the granuloma. **(a)** Bilateral vocal cord granuloma. **(b)** Vocal cord granuloma on the left side (courtesy of Dr. Yılmaz)

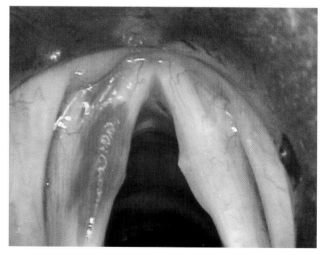

Fig. 3.6.9 Acute hemorrhagic lesion on the superior surface of the left vocal cord. Hemorrhage of the vocal cords generally occurs after shouting or singing. Usually one vocal cord is involved. The bleeding is into the lamina propria. Sudden onset of hoarseness after shouting is the classic anamnesis. Voice rest is recommended (courtesy of Dr. Yılmaz)

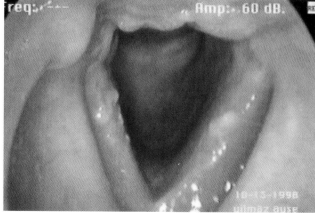

Fig. 3.6.11 Chronic laryngitis. The vocal cords are hyperemic and edematous. In long-standing laryngitis the epithelium is hypertrophic. Due to hypertrophy, irregularities may be seen at the free margin of the vocal cords. Epithelial changes are generally due to chronic vocal abuse and long-term smoking. Patients with hoarseness lasting longer than 6 weeks should be evaluated in detail and laryngeal carcinoma should be ruled out. If necessary, biopsy should be undertaken (courtesy of Dr. Yılmaz)

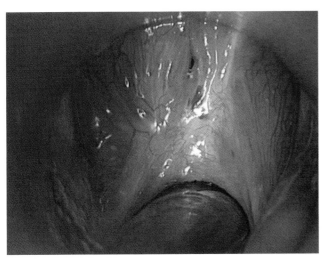

Fig. 3.6.12 Adhesion of the vocal cords at their middle third portion (courtesy of Dr. Yılmaz)

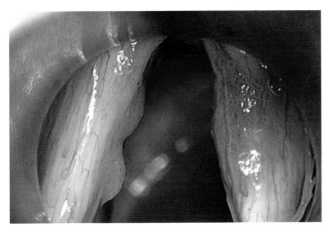

Fig. 3.6.13 Bilateral vocal cord papillomatous lesions in an adult patient (courtesy of Dr. Yılmaz)

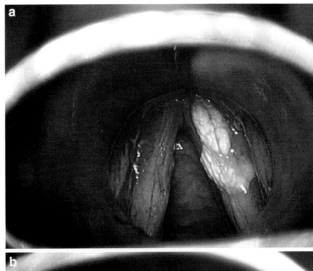

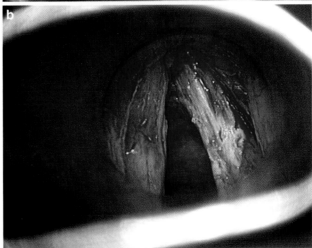

Fig. 3.6.15 (a) Leukoplakia of the right vocal cord. (b) After excision of the leukoplakia (courtesy of Dr. Yılmaz)

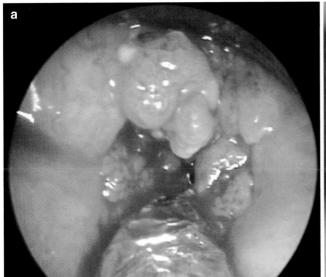

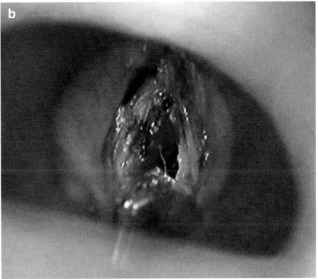

Fig. 3.6.14 (a) Juvenile laryngeal papillomatosis is the most common benign tumor of the larynx. It is caused by the human papilloma virus. The first symptom is hoarseness. When the lesion reaches an appropriate size for occlusion, stridor develops. CO_2 laser is of great help in the excision of papillomas. Many cases resolve by early adulthood. (b) After laser removal of the papilloma

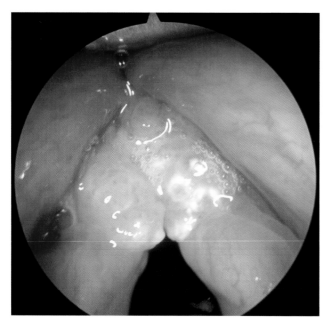

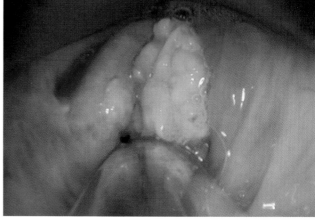

Fig. 3.6.17 Laryngeal carcinoma filling the glottis

Fig. 3.6.16 Vocal cord carcinoma located at the anterior commissure. Laryngeal carcinoma almost always occurs in smokers

3.7

Cysts

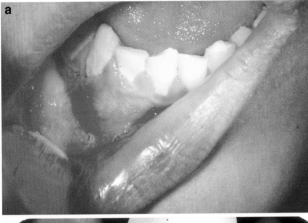

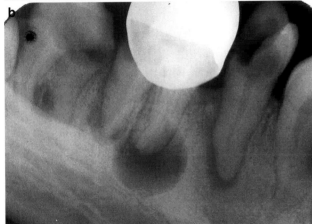

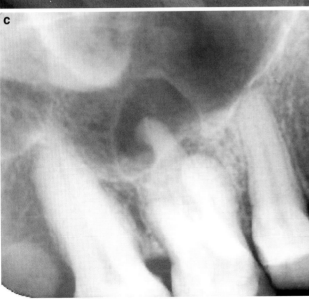

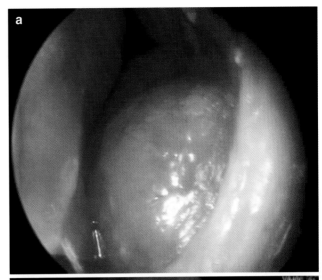

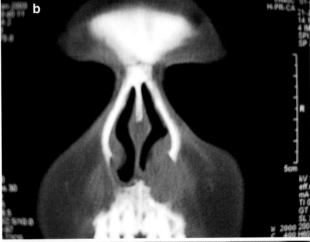

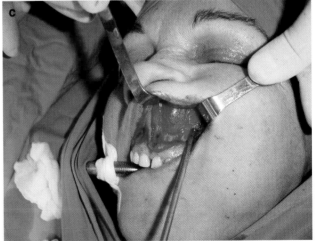

Fig. 3.7.1 (a–c) Radicular cysts (periapical cyst, dental cyst) are the most common odontogenic cysts, accounting for more than 50% of all odontogenic cysts. It starts with chronic tooth radix irritation. This irritation stimulates the epithelial remnants and forms a cystic structure. These cysts are often asymptomatic. If they become symptomatic, extraction of the tooth is necessary

Fig. 3.7.2 Nasolabial cysts (nasoalveolar cysts) are rare nonodontogenic developmental cysts. They generally occur as a unilateral swelling of the upper lip lateral to the midline and superficial to the maxilla. **(a)** Nasolabial cyst in the nasal vestibule. **(b)** Coronal CT image showing the nasopalatine cyst lateral to the midline and superficial to the maxilla. **(c)** Surgical exposure of the nasolabial cyst

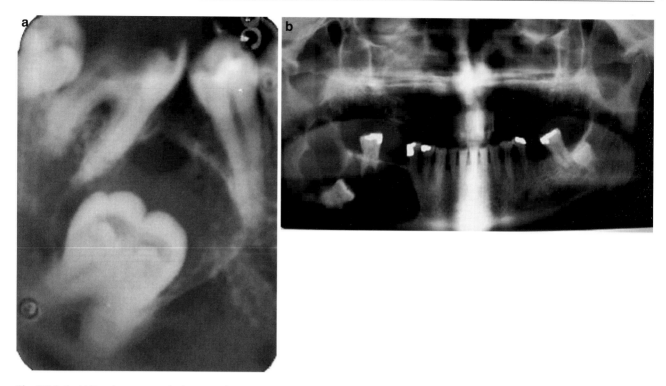

Fig. 3.7.3 (a, b) Dentigerous cyst is the second most common odontogenic cyst and is associated with an unerupted tooth, most commonly the impacted third mandibular or maxillary molars. On X-ray examination, a radiolucency surrounding a well-formed crown of an unerupted or impacted tooth is a characteristic finding. These cysts are generally asymptomatic (courtesy of Dr. Kansu)

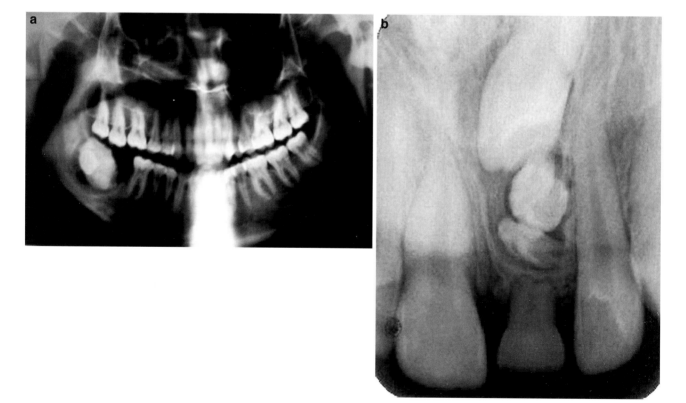

Fig. 3.7.4 (a) Odontoma is a hamartomatous malformation of the enamel organ. The majority of odontomas occur in the second and third molar area. Odontoma is more common in the mandible. On radiologic examination, irregular radiopacities surrounded by a narrow radiolucent band are seen. **(b)** Compound odontoma is the most differentiated type of odontogenic tumor. Multiple small teeth are seen on X-ray examination (courtesy of Dr. Kansu)

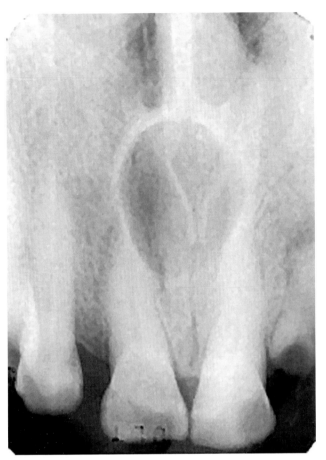

Fig. 3.7.5 Incisive canal cysts (nasopalatine cysts) are relatively common nonodontogenic developmental cysts. They occur in the palatal midline behind the maxillary central incisors in the region of the incisive canal

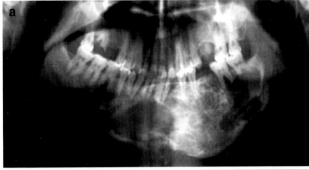

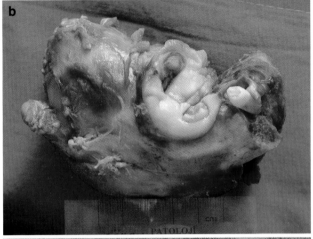

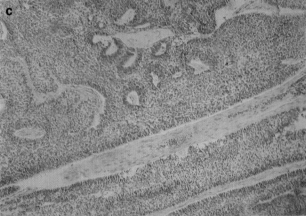

Fig. 3.7.6 Ameloblastomas most commonly occur in the age group of 20–50 years. The majority of tumors arise in the mandible (over 90%). (**a**) On X-ray examination, the typical soap bubble lucency in the mandible is characteristic of ameloblastoma. (**b**) Specimen after surgical excision. (**c**) Histologic picture of ameloblastoma, H&E, ×100. Cellular tumor composed of solid islands and basaloid cells at the periphery in the form of palisadic order

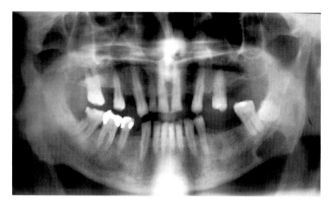

Fig. 3.7.7 Stafne bone cyst is not a real cyst, but a mandibular defect or depression on the lingual surface of the mandible. The cyst appears as an oval mass below the level of the mandibular canal near the angle of the mandible (courtesy of Dr. Kansu)

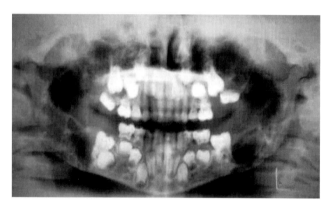

Fig. 3.7.8 Cherubism is an autosomal-dominant benign fibro-osseous disease of the jaws. The rami of the mandible are swollen. For this reason cherubism is also known as familial intraosseous swelling of the jaws. Clinically the face looks expanded in the area of the rami mandibulae. On X-ray, multilocular radiolucent areas are seen. Cherubism occurs between the ages of 2 and 20 years. It usually starts in the rami of the mandible bilaterally. At puberty the lesion begins to regress (courtesy of Dr. Kansu)

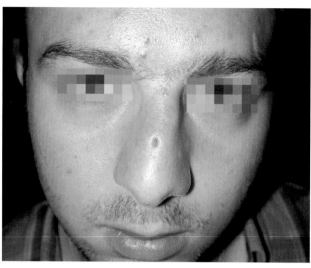

Fig. 3.7.9 Dermoid cyst. A cystic swelling is generally present at the glabella. There is a sinus commonly connecting the cyst to a punctum on the skin near the nasal tip. Extension of the cyst may go as far as the cribriform plate deep to the nasal bones

3.8

Salivary Gland Tumors

Salivary neoplasms may occur in all salivary glands. The majority of neoplasms (80%) occur in the parotid gland. The incidence of malignancy is highest in the sublingual glands (90%).

Pleomorphic adenomas mainly occur in the parotid glands. The tumor does not have a real capsule. It may have fingerlike extensions, and therefore enucleation of the tumor may result in a high recurrence rate. The surgical treatment of choice is parotidectomy. Since the facial nerve passes through the parotid gland, tumors of the parotid gland generally have a close relationship to the facial nerve. After identification of the facial nerve, the superficial lobe is dissected off the facial nerve. The tumors originate from the superficial lobe in 90% of cases. In these cases superficial parotidectomy should be performed. In 10% of cases the tumor may originate from the deep lobe. In these tumors originating from the deep lobe of the parotid gland, total parotidectomy should be performed and the surgery is much more difficult.

It is difficult to differentiate benign tumors from malignant ones. However, rapidly growing masses showing infiltration to the neighboring tissues or skin or causing facial nerve paralysis should be considered as malignant. Incisional biopsies cause tumor seeding and should not be performed.

Warthin tumor is only seen in male subjects and they are located at the tail of the gland and are frequently bilateral.

Table 3.8.1 Incidence of neoplasms in salivary glands

Salivary gland	Incidence (%)
Parotid gland	80
Submandibular gland	10
Minor salivary glands	9
Sublingual glands	1

Table 3.8.2 Salivary glands and the incidence of malignancy

Salivary gland	Incidence of malignancy (%)
Parotid gland	20
Submandibular gland	50
Minor salivary glands	50
Sublingual glands	90

Table 3.8.3 Classification of salivary gland neoplasms

Classification	Tumor
Benign	Pleomorphic adenoma Monomorphic adenomas (Warthin tumors etc.)
Malignant	Mucoepidermoid carcinoma Adenoid cystic carcinoma Acinic cell carcinoma Squamous cell carcinoma Adenocarcinoma Carcinoma ex pleomorphic adenoma Lymphoma Sarcoma

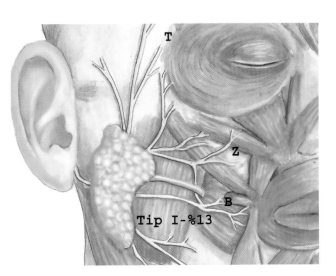

Fig. 3.8.1 The facial nerve passes through the parotid gland. Tumors of the parotid gland generally have a close relationship to the facial nerve. Therefore, facial nerve monitoring may help the surgeon avoid trauma to the facial nerve

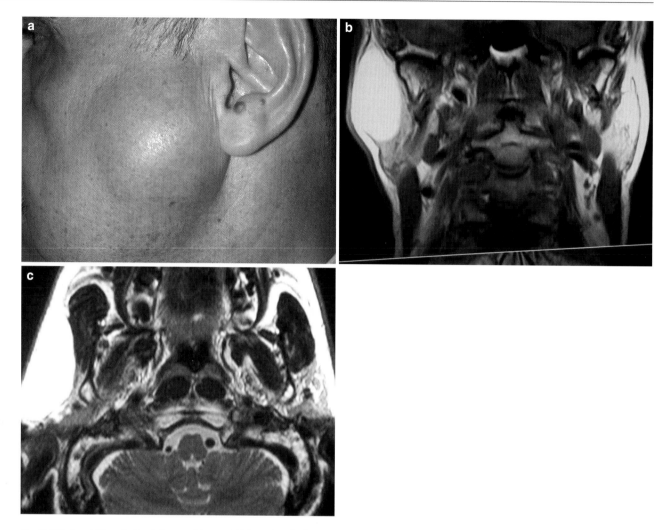

Fig. 3.8.2 (a–c) Mass in the left parotid area. MR imaging findings are typical for lipoma

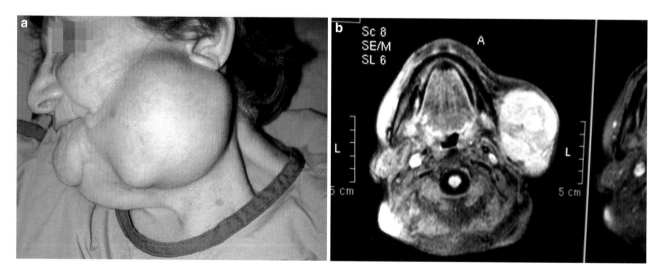

Fig. 3.8.3 (a) Benign parotid tumor on the left side. **(b)** Axial MR image shows tumor in the left parotid area (the pathology was reported as pleomorphic adenoma)

Fig. 3.8.4 Malignant parotid gland tumor invading the skin

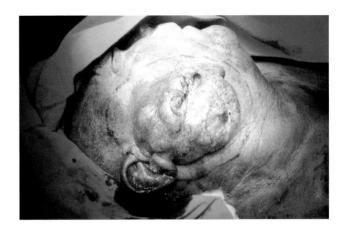

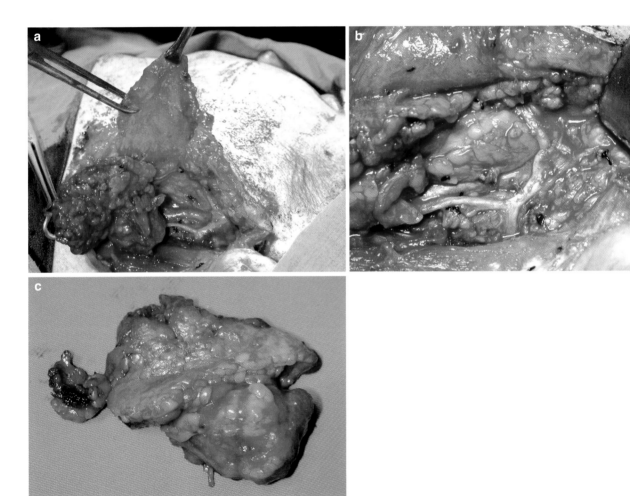

Fig. 3.8.5 Superficial parotidectomy. (**a**) The superficial lobe of the parotid gland is dissected from the facial nerve. (**b**) Facial nerve after dissection of the tumor. (**c**) Surgical specimen

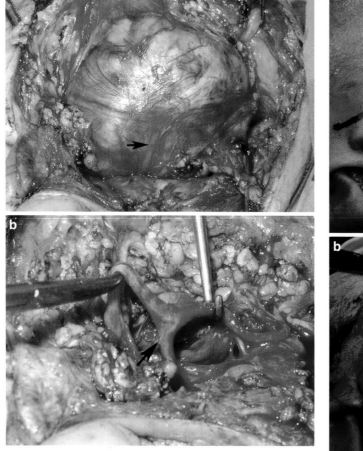

Fig. 3.8.6 (**a**) Parotid gland tumor located in the deep lobe and pushing the facial nerve laterally; *arrow* shows the facial nerve truncus. (**b**) After excision of the tumor, the facial nerve (black arrow) and its branches are seen (courtesy of TESAV)

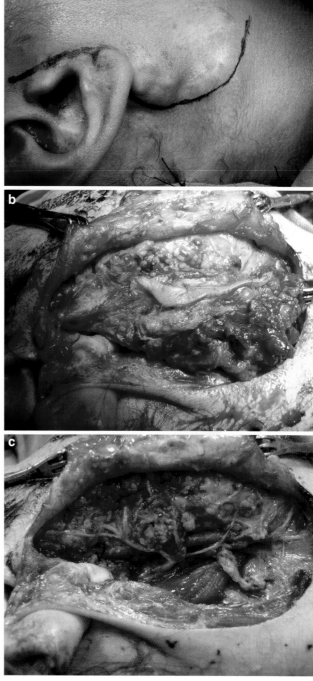

Fig. 3.8.7 Recurrent pleomorphic adenoma. Previous operation was enucleation of the pleomorphic adenoma. (**a**) Nodular masses of recurrent pleomorphic adenoma. (**b**) The previous skin incision is included in the specimen. (**c**) Facial nerve after parotidectomy (courtesy of Dr. Ünal)

3.9

Oral Cavity

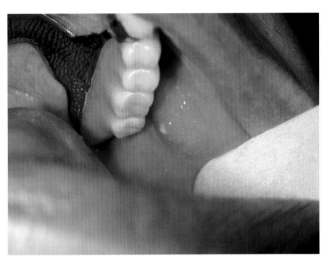

Fig. 3.9.1 Acute parotitis. Purulent material is draining out through the Stenson duct on applying pressure to the parotid gland

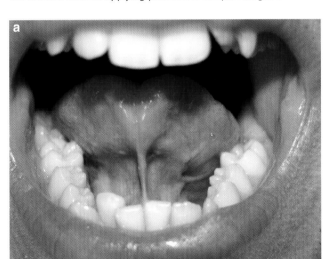

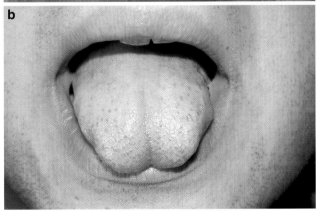

Fig. 3.9.2 (a, b) Tongue tie. This is indeed a short frenulum linguae preventing the patient from protruding the tongue. It does not cause any symptoms. Division of the frenulum can easily be performed

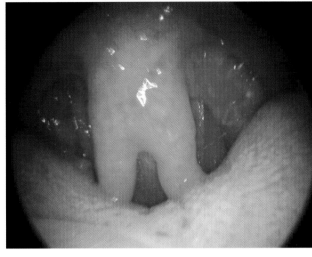

Fig. 3.9.3 Bifid uvula is a congenital deformity of the palate. It has no clinical significance and does not require any treatment. Sometimes a submucosal cleft palate may be associated with the deformity

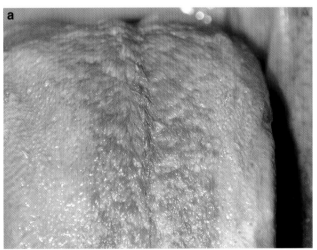

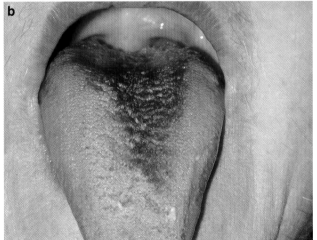

Fig. 3.9.4 (a, b) Hairy tongue. This is due to hypertrophy of the filiform papillae. Tobacco use is generally the cause. Cleaning the tongue with a soft toothbrush may help improve the appearance. Stopping smoking is the most important factor

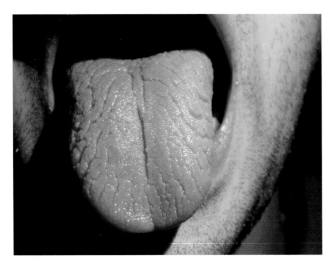

Fig. 3.9.5 Fissured tongue has no clinical significance. If it is associated with recurrent episodes of facial nerve paralysis and upper lip edema it is called Melkersson-Rosenthal syndrome

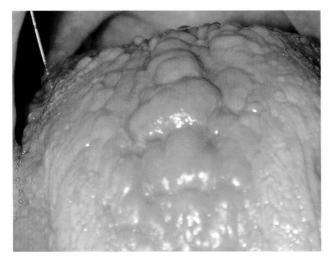

Fig. 3.9.6 Median rhomboid glossitis is a histologically benign pathology and is not truly glossitis. The lesion is characterized by nodular elevated areas devoid of papillae located anterior to the circumvallate papillae on the dorsum of the tongue

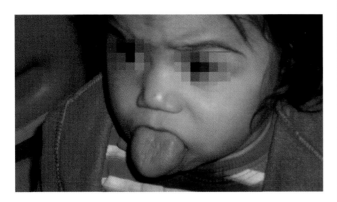

Fig. 3.9.7 Macroglossia. An enlarged tongue is generally not symptomatic. It may very rarely cause abnormal speech. In the adult, macroglossia may be associated with amyloidosis. In children, lymphangioma may be the cause

a

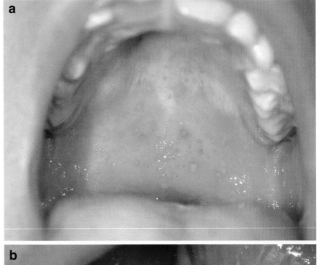

b

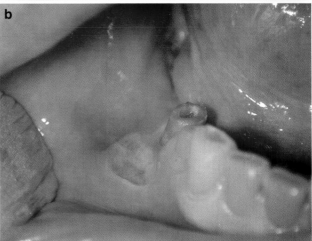

Fig. 3.9.8 (**a**) Herpes stomatitis is caused by herpes simplex virus. The small, painful lesions have red margins around them. In contrast to aphthous lesions there is a bad smell and increased salivation. (**b**) Aphthous stomatitis is the most common cause of ulcers in the oral cavity. They have similar clinical features to herpes simplex eruptions, but herpes simplex eruptions involve the hard palate more often. The etiology is unknown, although vitamin B, folic acid, and iron deficiencies have been implicated

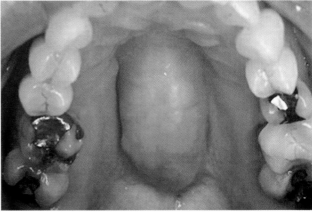

Fig. 3.9.9 Torus palatinus is a nodular or lobular bony growth in the midline of the hard palate covered by normal mucosa. Treatment is surgical removal (courtesy of Dr. Hersek)

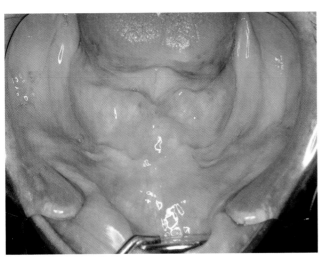

Fig. 3.9.10 The mandible has been resorbed due to wearing dentures for a long period of time (courtesy of Dr. Hersek)

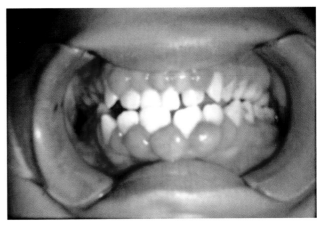

Fig. 3.9.13 Hypertrophic gingivitis. Overgrowth of the gingiva surrounding the base of the teeth may sometimes cover the teeth. Vitamin deficiencies and hematopoietic diseases should be ruled out

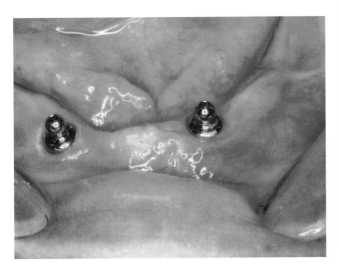

Fig. 3.9.11 Dental implants in an edentulous patient (courtesy of Dr. Hersek)

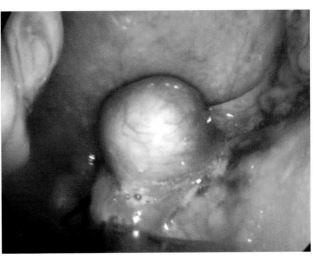

Fig. 3.9.14 Mucous cyst at the tongue base

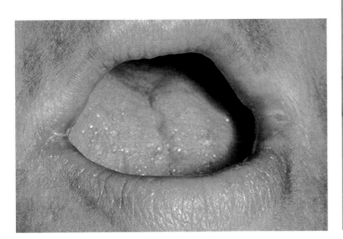

Fig. 3.9.12 Angular cheilitis may be due to iron deficiency or vitamin B deficiency. *Staphylococcus aureus* and *Candida* infections may be predisposing factors (courtesy of Dr. Hersek)

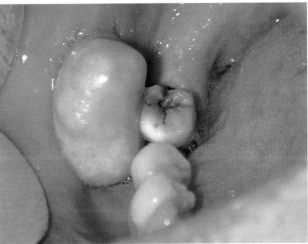

Fig. 3.9.15 Fibroma of the buccal mucosa. This is a benign lesion and is generally due to dental trauma. Treatment consists of eliminating the trauma and excising the lesion

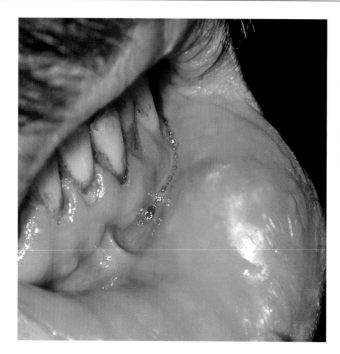

Fig. 3.9.16 Mucocele of the lip. A mucocele is a cystic, nontender swelling. It is either due to occlusion of the duct of a mucous gland or due to extravasation of mucus from a mucous gland into the surrounding tissue. Treatment is by simple excision

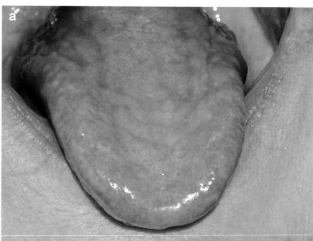

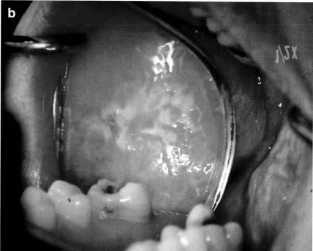

Fig. 3.9.18 Lichen planus. **(a)** Tongue, **(b)** buccal mucosa. The most common form in the oral cavity is the reticular form located on the buccal mucosa. It originates in the posterior area and spreads anteriorly. Lichen planus may present as a fine lacework of white reticular hyperkeratotic papules or annular lesions on the dorsum of the tongue. It is a self-limited disease. Sometimes topical steroid ointments may be required

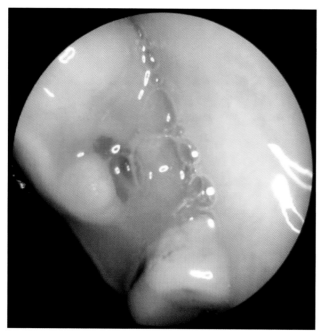

Fig. 3.9.17 Oroantral fistula. The root of molar teeth sometimes may extend into the maxillary sinus cavity. Extractions of these molar teeth may lead to a fistula between the oral cavity and maxillary sinus

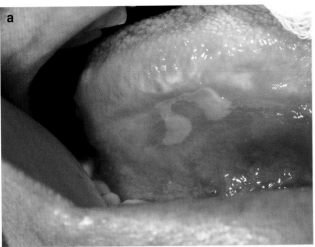

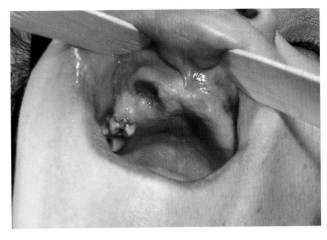

Fig. 3.9.21 Fibro-osseous lesions may cause significant bone destruction

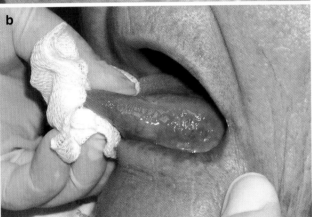

Fig. 3.9.19 (a, b) Leukoplakia is a white lesion. It is due to increased production of keratin and thickening of the epithelial layer

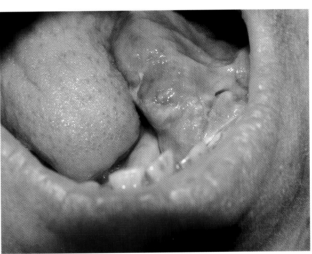

Fig. 3.9.22 Giant cell granuloma of the jaws occurs most frequently in female patients under 30 years of age and the majority of the lesions are found in the mandible

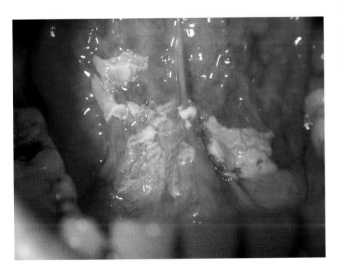

Fig. 3.9.20 Leukoplakia located on the floor of the mouth. Excision of the lesion should be performed due to the risk of malignant transformation

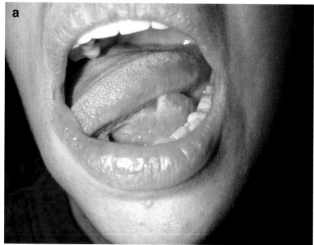

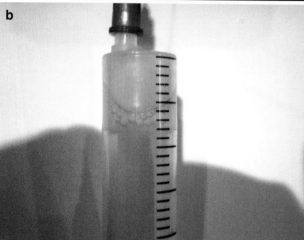

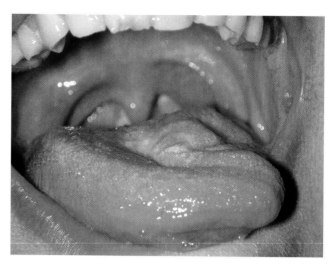

Fig. 3.9.25 Atrophy on the left side of the tongue following 12th nerve paralysis. Tongue is pushed to the paralyzed side

Fig. 3.9.23 (a, b) The ranula is a mucocele originating from the sublingual salivary glands. It is a cystic structure. Inside the ranula there is yellow fluid which can be drained easily. It occupies the floor of the mouth. Total surgical excision is not always possible due to the very thin wall of the mucocele. Marsupialization is also an adequate treatment method that can be used

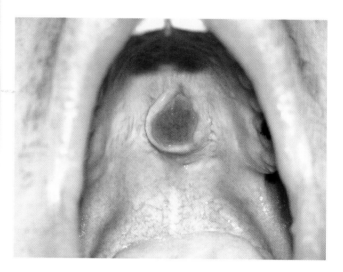

Fig. 3.9.26 Minor salivary gland tumor, pleomorphic adenoma of the hard palate, after biopsy. A palatal swelling may be due to a tumor of the minor salivary glands. Generally they are benign tumors. Other malignant tumors may also be considered. Diagnosis is made by biopsy

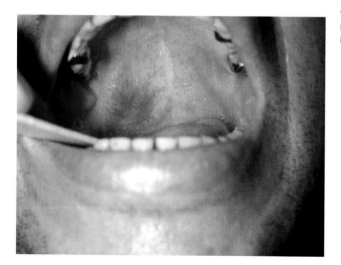

Fig. 3.9.24 Hemangioma on the left side of the palate

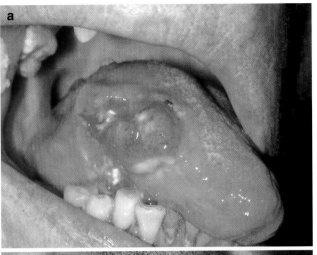

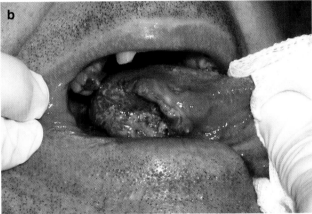

Fig. 3.9.27 (a, b) Various squamous cell carcinomas of the tongue. Generally occurs at the lateral edge of the tongue. Diagnosis is made by biopsy. Treatment is partial glossectomy with a neck dissection and radiotherapy

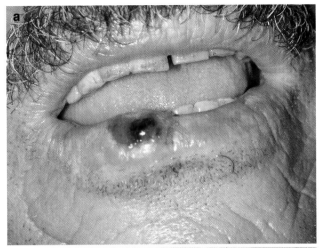

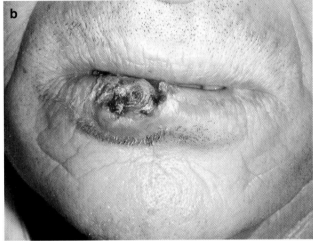

Fig. 3.9.29 (a, b) Lower lip carcinoma

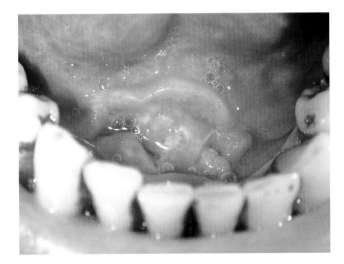

Fig. 3.9.28 Squamous cell carcinoma of the floor of the mouth

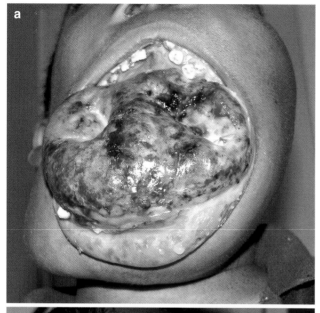

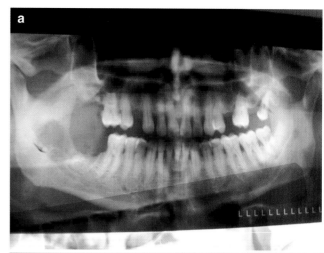

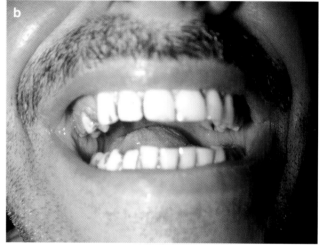

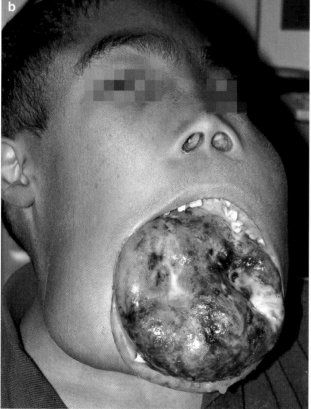

Fig. 3.9.31 **(a)** Squamous cell carcinoma of the retromolar trigone causing destruction of the mandible. **(b)** Invasion of the pterygoid muscles causes trismus

Fig. 3.9.30 **(a, b)** Squamous cell carcinoma which fills the oral cavity and prevents normal functions (Courtesy of TESAV)

3.10

Neck Masses

Thyroglossal Duct Cyst

The most common congenital neck mass in children is a thyroglossal duct cyst. Thyroglossal duct cysts are most commonly located below the hyoid bone; however, they may be found anywhere between the base of the tongue and the superior border of the thyroid gland. They move on swallowing and on tongue protrusion. Unless infected they are asymptomatic. The patient only complains about a lump in the neck. Treatment is complete excision of both the cyst and the entire thyroglossal duct up to the foramen cecum at the base of the tongue. Therefore, it is necessary to remove the central portion of the hyoid bone.

Dermoid Cyst

Dermoid cysts are usually located in the submental region in the midline. They are epithelial remnants occurring along the lines of fusion in the embryo. Dermoids are lined by epidermis and may contain hair follicles, epidermis, and sebaceous glands. Dermoid cysts should be excised.

Branchial Arch Anomalies

Branchial arch anomalies (sinuses, fistulas, cysts) result from abnormalities in the normal development of the branchial apparatus. They are present at birth but usually present in the second or third decade of life.

First Branchial Cleft Anomalies

First branchial arch anomalies are not so common. These anomalies are commonly found at the angle of the mandible, and a fistula or sinus tract opens into the external auditory canal at the bony cartilaginous junction. First branchial cleft anomalies are duplications of both the membranous and bony external canal. Their course may pass above or below the facial nerve.

Second Branchial Cleft Anomalies

Second branchial cleft anomalies are the most common branchial defects. They have an opening in the lower half of the neck and their course is along the anterior border of the sternocleidomastoid muscle. They open in the tonsillar fossa. They are lateral to the structures in the neck.

Laryngoceles

Laryngoceles are dilations of the saccule, the lateral end of the ventricle, and are caused by increased intralaryngeal pressures. They may be classified as external or internal according to their relationship to the laryngeal cartilages. Internal laryngoceles are within the endolarynx, and they lie medial to the laryngeal cartilage. External laryngoceles extend outside the larynx through the thyrohyoid membrane, generally at the point where the superior laryngeal nerve passes. The treatment is surgical excision if they are symptomatic.

Cystic Hygromas

Cystic hygromas are anomalies of the lymph channels. Fifty percent present by 1 year of age, and 90% by age 2. They are soft, irregular swellings. They may be located in the floor of mouth or in the lateral neck area. Treatment is surgical excision. Surgery may be postponed until the child is 3–4 years of age, because of the possibility of involution and the relative technical easiness of the surgery at an older age if there is no risk of airway compromise or rapid growth.

Hemangiomas

Hemangiomas are benign tumors that are seen in the neonatal period. Spontaneous regression may occur as the child grows.

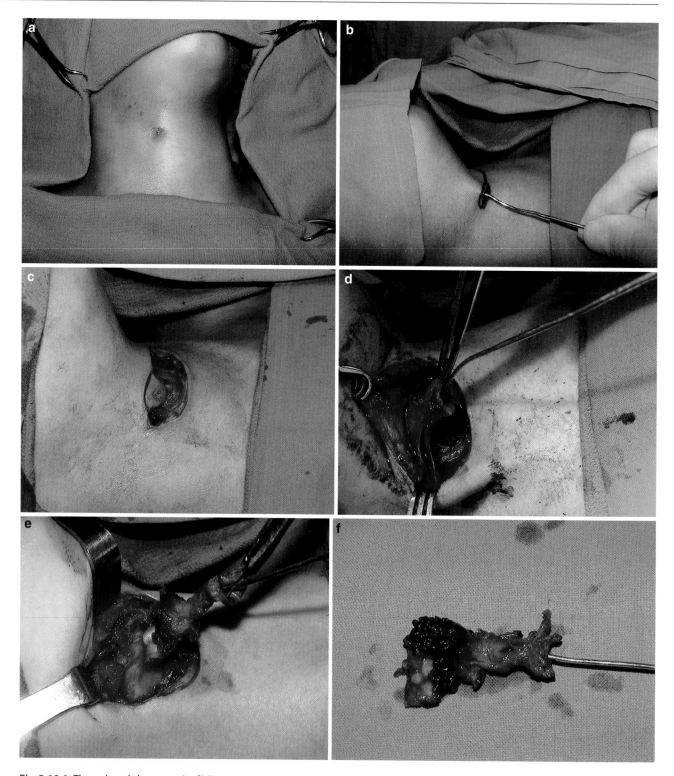

Fig. 3.10.1 Thyroglossal duct cyst. (**a–f**) Treatment is complete excision of both the cyst and the entire thyroglossal duct up to the foramen cecum at the base of the tongue. Removal of the central portion of the hyoid bone is mandatory to prevent recurrences (courtesy of Dr. Unal)

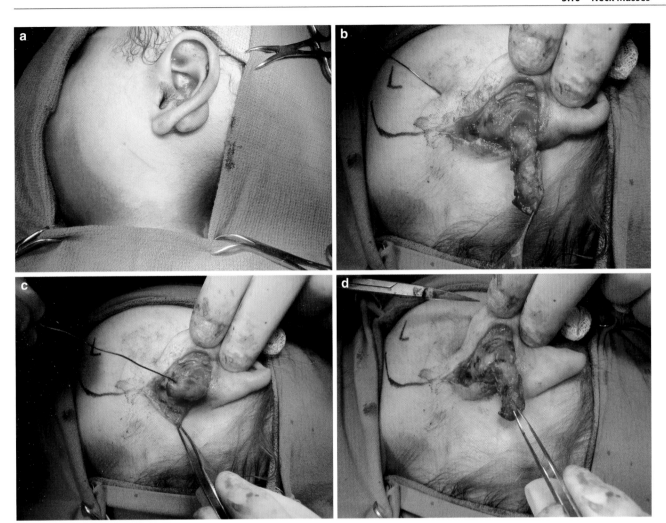

Fig. 3.10.2 (a–d) First branchial cleft anomalies are commonly found at the angle of the mandible. A fistula or sinus tract opens into the external auditory canal at the bony cartilaginous junction. First branchial cleft anomalies are duplications of both the membranous and bony external canal. Their course may pass above or below the facial nerve (courtesy of Dr. Unal)

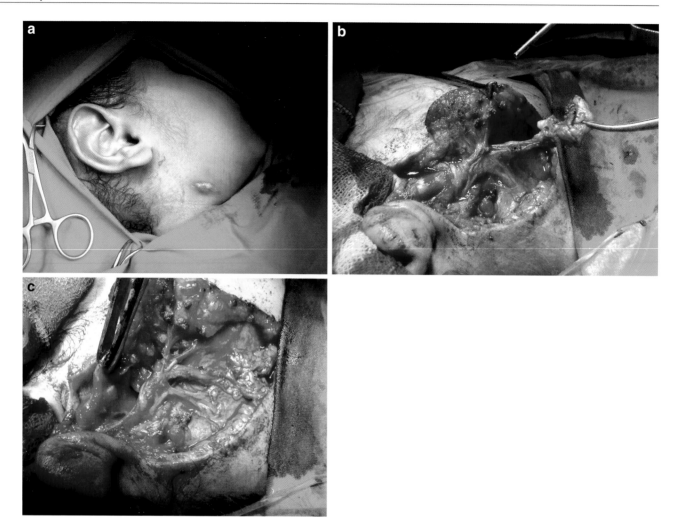

Fig. 3.10.3 (a–c) First branchial cleft anomaly. Its course passes below the facial nerve and the sinus tract opens into the external auditory canal at the bony cartilaginous junction (courtesy of Dr. Unal)

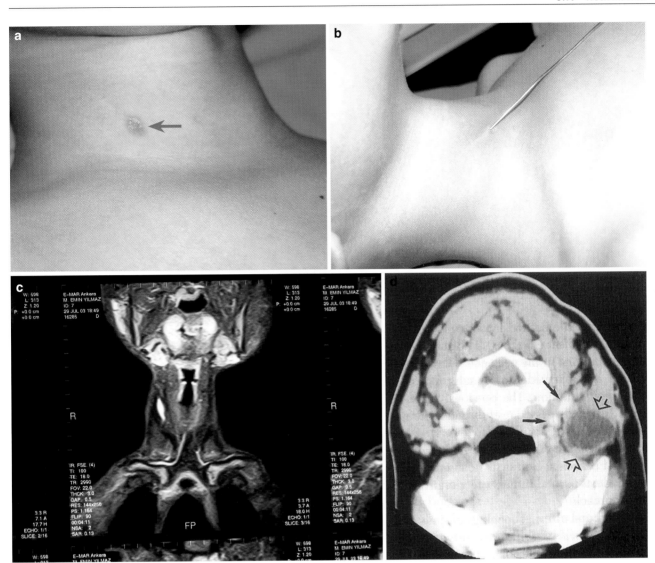

Fig. 3.10.4 (a-d) Second branchial cleft anomaly. These anomalies have an opening in the lower half of the neck (red arrow) and their course is along the anterior border of the sternocleidomastoid muscle. They open in the tonsillar fossa. They are lateral to the structures in the neck. Sometimes the cystic portion may present as a lateral neck mass (arrows) (courtesy of Dr. Unal)

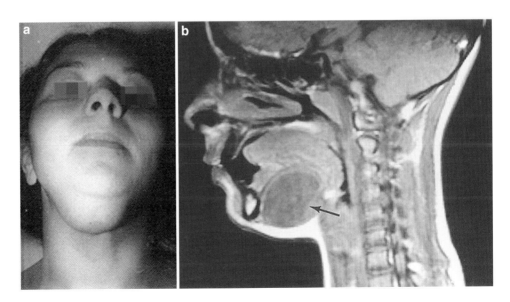

Fig. 3.10.5 (a, b) Dermoid cysts are usually located in the submental region in the midline

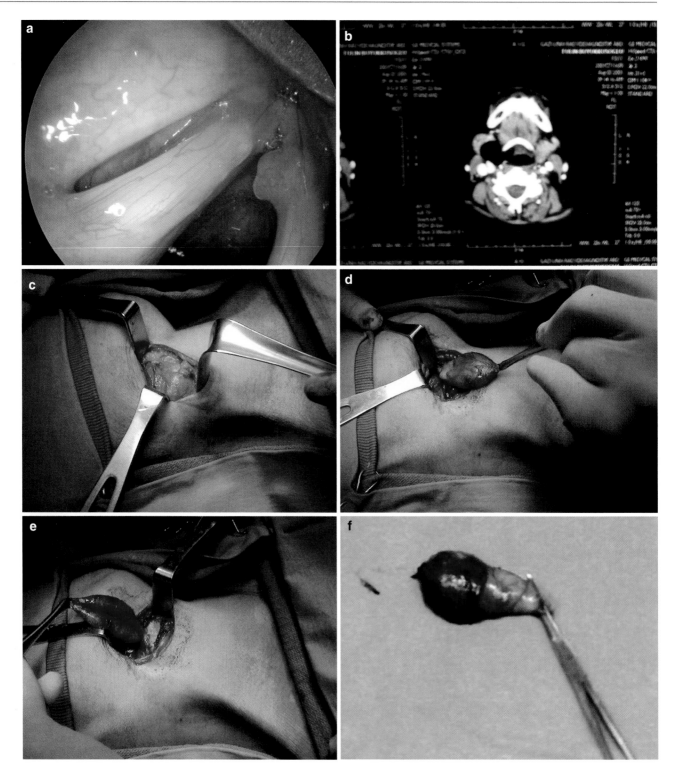

Fig. 3.10.6 (a–f) Laryngoceles are dilations of the saccule, the lateral end of the ventricle, and are caused by increased intralaryngeal pressures. External laryngoceles extend outside the larynx through the thyrohyoid membrane, generally at the point where the superior laryngeal nerve passes. Treatment is surgical excision if they are symptomatic (courtesy of Dr. Unal)

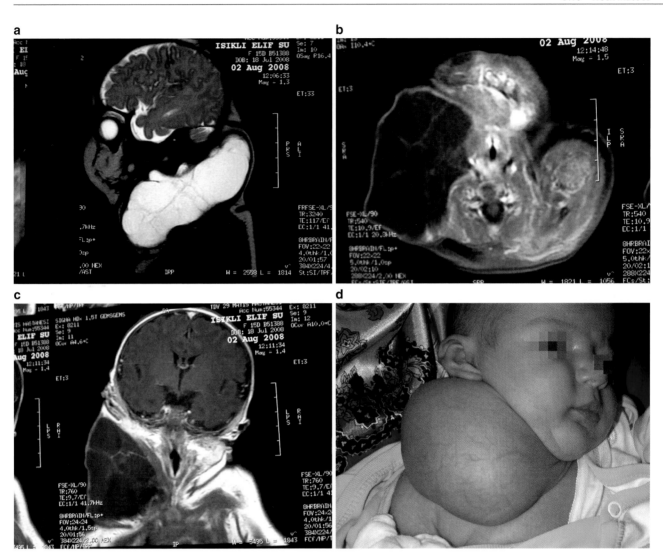

Fig. 3.10.7 (a–d) Cystic hygromas are soft, irregular swellings. They may be located in the floor of mouth or in the lateral neck area

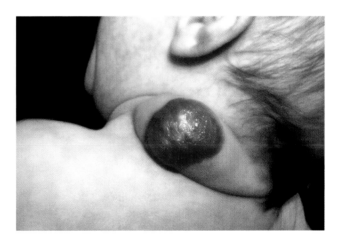

Fig. 3.10.8 Hemangiomas are benign tumors that are seen in the neonatal period

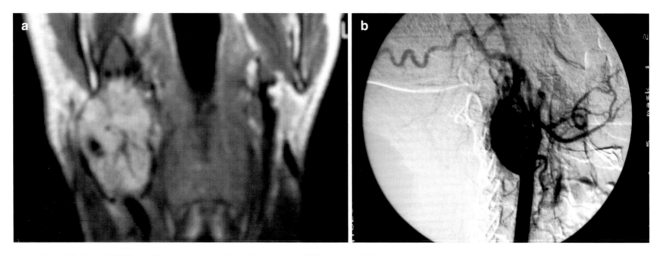

Fig. 3.10.9 (a, b) Carotid body tumor. Carotid body tumors arise from the carotid body located at the bifurcation of the internal carotid artery. Pulsation may be palpated and a bruit can be heard by stethoscope. The tumor can be moved in the horizontal plane but not in the vertical plane. On MR examination, the highly vascularized tumor located between the external and internal carotid arteries confirms the diagnosis

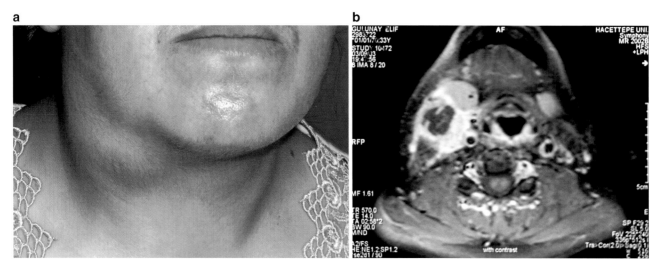

Fig. 3.10.10 (a, b) Tuberculosis. Cervical lymph node enlargement due to tuberculosis is not common but is becoming more frequent. Due to the chronicity of the disease they may be confused with neoplasms, especially lymphomas. They are multiple and coalesce. Pulmonary tuberculosis may associated with tuberculous lymphadenopathy. Node biopsy, if necessary for histological confirmation, should always be excisional. Incisional biopsy may result in fistula and chronic discharge

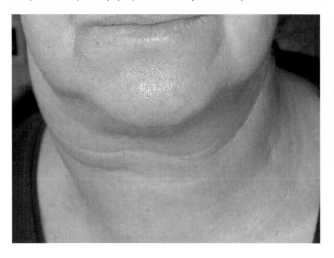

Fig. 3.10.11 Very large lymphadenopathy located at the right upper neck in a patient with lymphoma

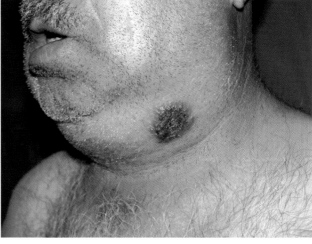

Fig. 3.10.12 Deep neck infection

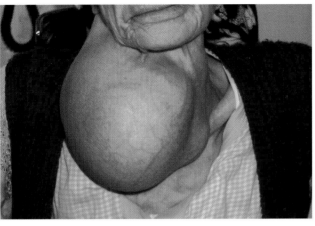

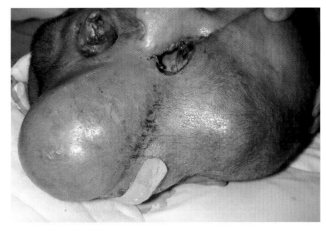

Fig. 3.10.13 Anaplastic thyroid carcinoma (courtesy of Dr. Ş. Hosal)

Fig. 3.10.14 Recurrent giant malignant fibrosarcoma on the left side of the face

EAR NOSE

THROAT AND NECK

3.11

Neck Malignancies

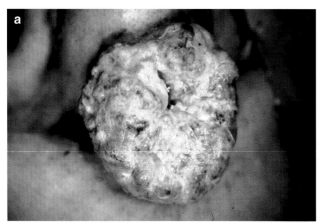

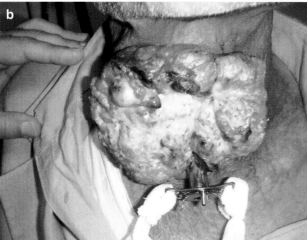

Fig. 3.11.1 (a) Peristomal recurrence that developed at the site of tracheotomy in a patient with laryngeal carcinoma with subglottic extension. **(b)** Recurrent laryngeal carcinoma with skin invasion causing respiratory obstruction

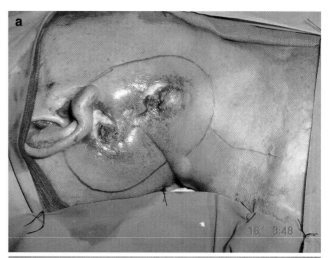

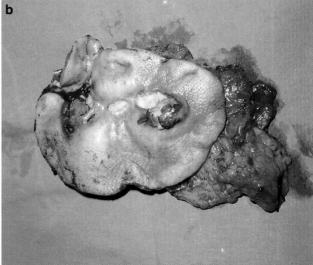

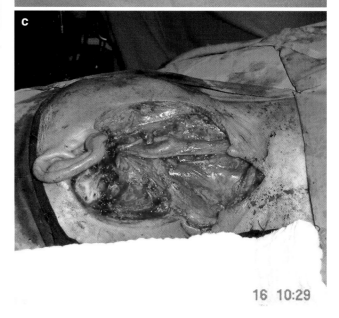

Fig. 3.11.2 (a) Recurrence of a malignant tumor that invaded the skin in the neck. **(b)** Specimen after excision of the lesion. **(c)** The defect in the neck after excision of the lesion. Common, internal, and external carotid arteries, vagus nerve, and hypoglossal nerve crossing these structures are seen

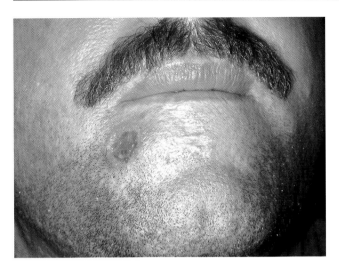

Fig. 3.11.3 Recurrent lower lip carcinoma

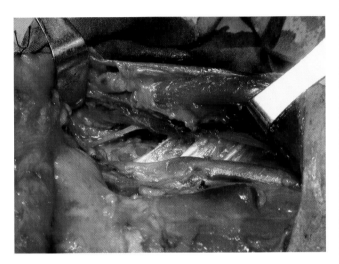

Fig. 3.11.5 Neck dissection. Behind the retracted sternocleidomastoid muscle, the 11th nerve in the upper triangle and cutaneous sensory nerves of the neck in the lower half are seen

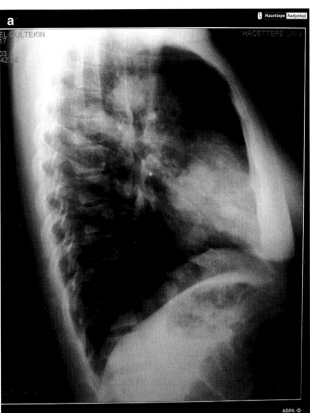

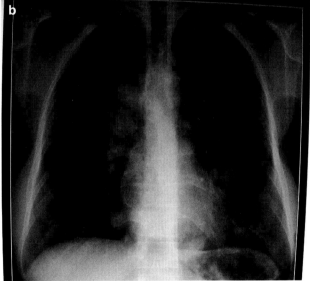

Fig. 3.11.4 (a, b) Pulmonary metastasis in a patient with head and neck carcinoma

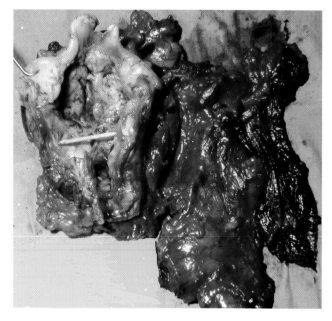

Fig. 3.11.6 Total laryngectomy and unilateral radical neck dissection

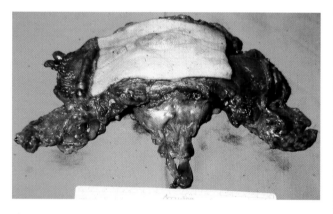

Fig. 3.11.7 A recurrent laryngeal carcinoma with skin invasion. Total laryngectomy with bilateral radical neck dissection and bilateral paratracheal and retrosternal dissection were performed. The neck skin was included in the specimen

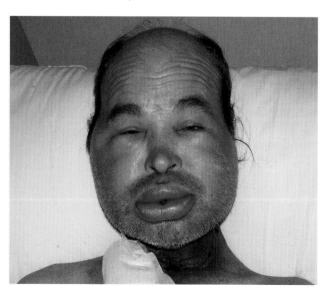

Fig. 3.11.8 Edema of the face in a patient after bilateral radical neck dissection

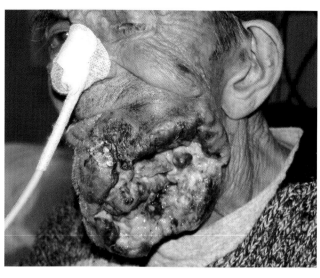

Fig. 3.11.9 Squamous cell carcinoma which destroyed the mandible

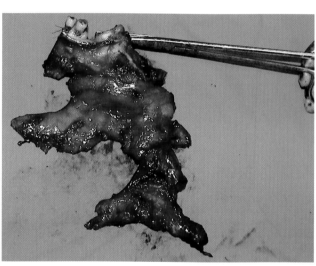

Fig. 3.11.10 Segmental mandibular resection with bilateral neck dissection due to carcinoma of the floor of the mouth

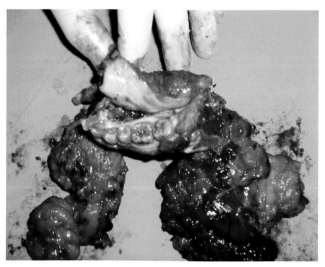

Fig. 3.11.11 Carcinoma of the floor of the oral cavity. Partial mandibular resection with bilateral neck dissection was performed (courtesy of Dr. Ş. Hosal)

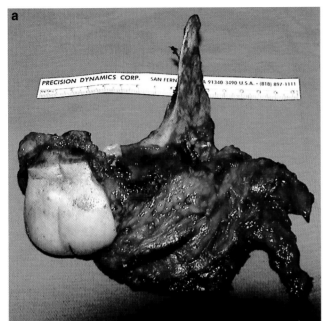

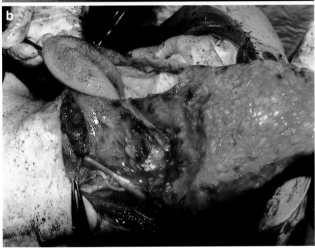

Fig. 3.11.12 (a) Hemimandibulectomy with unilateral neck dissection. The skin of the mentum has been included in the specimen. **(b)** Defect in the neck after resection of the lesion

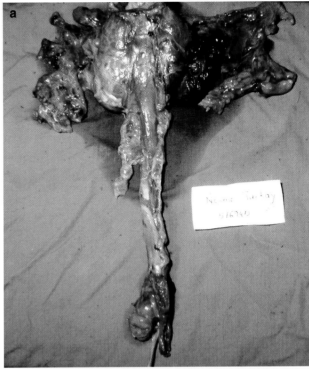

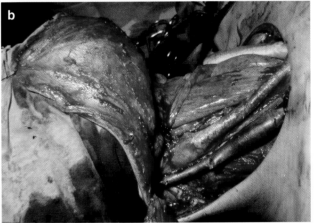

Fig. 3.11.14 (a) Total laryngopharyngo-osephagectomy with bilateral functional neck dissection. **(b)** Reconstruction by gastric pull-up

The development of new reconstructive techniques has facilitated more aggressive surgical procedures. They can be used to resurface large skin or mucosal defects and to provide coverage for major vascular structures. Besides local and pedicled myocutaneous flaps, free flaps help the surgeon overcome difficulties such as limited arc of rotation, tension at the edges, bulky skin paddles, and donor site morbidity.

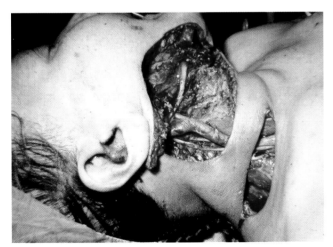

Fig. 3.11.13 Hemimandibulectomy with unilateral radical neck dissection via a McFee incision

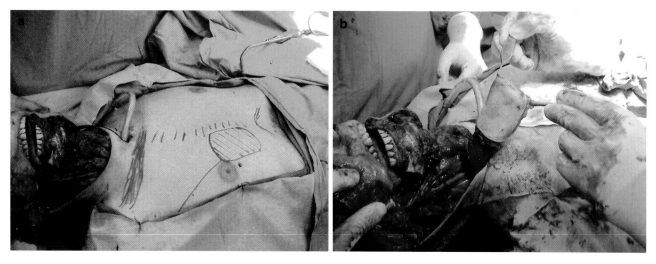

Fig. 3.11.15 (a) Preparation of the pectoralis major flap. (b) Pectoralis major flap with its skin pad (courtesy of Dr. Ş. Hosal)

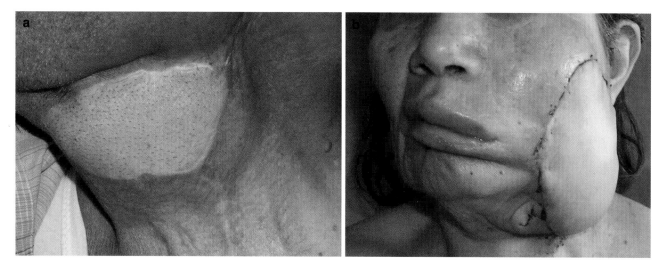

Fig. 3.11.16 Pectoralis major flap for reconstruction of a large defect (a) in the neck and (b) in the face (courtesy of Dr. Ş. Hosal)

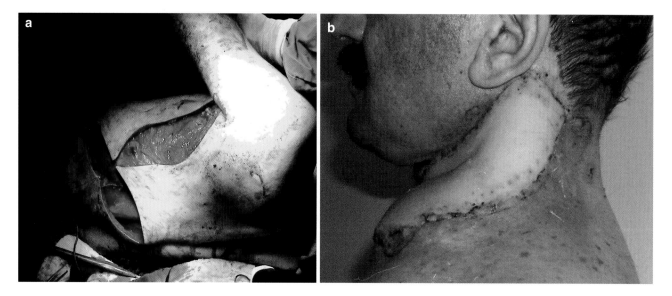

Fig. 3.11.17 (a, b) Closure of a defect in the neck with latissimus dorsi flap (courtesy of Dr. Ş. Hosal)

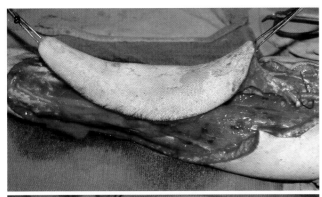

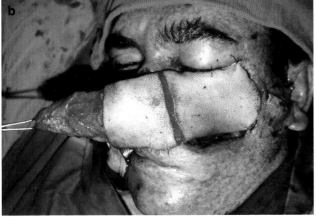

Fig. 3.11.18 Radial forearm free flap. **(a)** Preparation and **(b)** closure of the defect in the face (courtesy of Dr. Ş. Hosal)

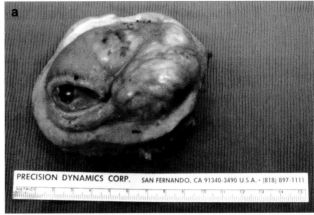

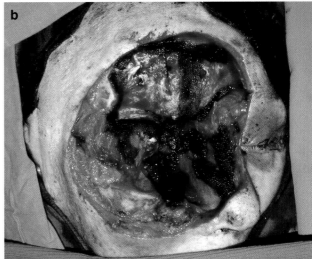

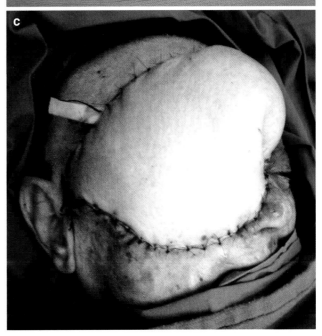

Fig. 3.11.19 Excision of squamous cell carcinoma in the right eye and forehead area. **(a)** The specimen, **(b)** the defect, and **(c)** closure by a rectus abdominis free flap (courtesy of Dr. Ş. Hosal)

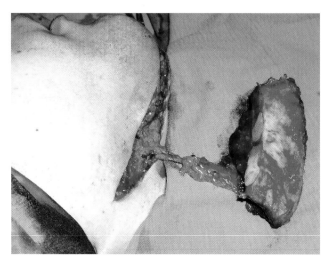

Fig. 3.11.20 Free bone graft prepared from iliac crest for reconstruction of a mandibular bony defect (courtesy of Dr. Ş. Hosal)

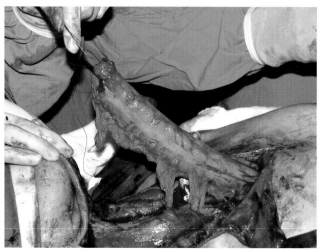

Fig. 3.11.21 Reconstruction of the esophagus with a free jejunal flap

Index

Printing and Binding: Stürtz GmbH, Würzburg